STRANGE KINDNESS

Mabel S. Chu Tow
Melissa Ann (Mei An) Reed

Hamilton Books
A member of
The Rowman & Littlefield Publishing Group
Lanham · Boulder · New York · Toronto · Plymouth, UK

Copyright © 2008 by
Hamilton Books
4501 Forbes Boulevard
Suite 200
Lanham, Maryland 20706
Hamilton Books Acquisitions Department (301) 459-3366

Estover Road
Plymouth PL6 7PY
United Kingdom

Library of Congress Control Number: 2007933223
ISBN-13: 978-0-7618-3881-4 (paperback : alk. paper)
ISBN-10: 0-7618-3881-3 (paperback : alk. paper)

*A good teacher for a day
is like a parent for a lifetime.*

-Chinese Proverb

CONTENTS

FOREWORD

Kindness
   by Naomi Shihab Nye

Before you know what kindness really is
you must lose things,
feel the future dissolve in a moment
like salt in a weakened broth.
What you held in your hand,
what you counted and carefully saved,
all this must go so you know
how desolate the landscape can be
between the regions of kindness.
How you ride and ride
thinking the bus will never stop,
the passengers eating maize and chicken
will stare out the window forever.

Before you learn the tender gravity of kindness,
you must travel where the Indian in a white poncho
lies dead by the side of the road.
You must see how this could be you,
how he too was someone
who journeyed through the night with plans
and the simple breath that kept him alive.

Before you know kindness as the deepest thing inside,
you must know sorrow as the other deepest thing.
You must wake up with sorrow,
you must speak to it till your voice
catches the thread of all sorrows
and you see the size of the cloth.

Then it is only kindness that makes sense anymore,
only kindness that ties your shoes
and sends you out into the day to mail letters and purchase bread,
only kindness that raises its head
from the crowd of the world to say
It is I you have been looking for,
and then goes with you everywhere
like a shadow or a friend.

By permission of the author, Naomi Shihab Nye, 2006. From her collection of poems, *Words Under the Words*.

PREFACE

When Mabel (Chu, Cho Shin) Tow (1914–1999), one of the first Chinese women to practice medicine in China and the United States, shares her story with us, we may experience "the tender gravity of kindness," the generative transmission of her lineage. This story may say, in its own way, what the poet, William Stafford says in his last poem, ***Are You Mr. William Stafford?*** "You can't tell when strange things with meaning /will happen." This story also participates in the movement of *tikkun olam*, is an act of repairing the world.

Melissa Ann Reed, Ph.D.
Portland, Oregon
January 22, 2007

ACKNOWLEDGMENTS

May my deepest appreciation and gladness flow to all who have supported the making and the offering of *Strange Kindness*. More than an honor, the experience of working with Mabel S. Chu Tow, whose vision makes every life and every day sacred, was an undreamed of, unexpected joy. More than a privilege, the experience of working with Dr. Vay Liang William Go and the commentary authors, each of whom made time to add a new dimension and a new author-reader relationship to Tow's story, increased my faith. To each person who gave technical support in the preparation of the manuscript, Paula L. Smith-Vanderslice and Catherine Forrest Getzie of University Press of America, Ross Ludeman, and Debi Brimacombe, I am especially grateful. To the University Press of America editor, Patti Belcher, who gave me astute advice and kind support, increasing my hope and patience, I am dearly thankful. Warm thanks to my teacher, Wang, Gongyi, who tutored my experience of Chinese culture through the practices of Chinese calligraphy and brush painting, to Bill Allshouse, who inspired the painting for the book cover, to the lovely Inga Dubay, artist and calligrapher, who always weaves kindness into her art and life, and to special friends Joan and Don McMillan, Elizabeth Goeke, Jeffrey Cawley, and the Caritas Ministry at Trinity Episcopal Cathedral.

INTRODUCTION

In old China, friends would gather to share tea and write poems to honor one another. Mabel S. Chu Tow commemorates this custom in one of her untitled poems, concluding:

> We write our thoughts
> to enjoy them together,
> again and again,
> to remember our feelings—
>
> I think about my memories
> and this poem that will be
> forever like our friendship,
> always unfolding

In this same sacramental spirit of tea, friendship, and written word, Tow shares *Strange Kindness*, a reflection upon her life (1914–1999). One of the first Chinese women to practice medicine both in China and in the United States, Tow reflects upon her life by asking many questions—questions concerning whether she fulfilled her life's purpose, questions examining the roots and directions of her career path, questions wondering how she might honor the kindness of people who supported her profession of healing and faith. Her listener is always a friend within the sacred circle of tea, poem, and spoken word.

With her questions, Tow juxtaposes the choices, her own and others', which created her history and *gave her today.* She views questions and choices through a selected lens, the perspective beginning the discourse of *Strange Kindness*: "When you are young, you are good, but when you grow up, you choose your own nature." This Chinese proverb from *The Book of Three Word Chants* recognizes each person as a free artist of his or her own character and imparts the Taoist wisdom of change, a wisdom realized by Lewis Carroll's Alice of *Wonderland* when, in empathy with the caterpillar, she replies, "I know who I *was* when I woke up this morning, but I think I must have been changed several times since then."

Learned orally by generations of Chinese children, repeated by Tow, and then repeated and embodied silently by Tow's reader in the context of *Strange Kindness*, this chant moves speaker, listener, and reader into *tian ren he yi*, a condition of oneness with the universe. To be at one with the universe through the light of pure heartmind is the spiritual aim and holistic character of Classical Chinese Medicine, primarily a meditation practice as Tow learned it between the ages of four and fifteen from her father, Dr. Chu. CCM physicians discerned, through unitive consciousness, how to release and balance a patient's energy.

Through the looking glass of this ancient chant, then, Tow offers us her spiritual autobiography, the Self-overheard dialogues of her life. These dialogues aim to honor each individual whose ineffable kindness enabled her to fulfill her father's wish for her life. Weaving together these dialogues are Tow's introspective, Self-questioning dialogues, conversations with herself unfolding her deepest wonder: "Many people guided me in my life's way/ to follow in my father's footsteps. / Why? / I don't know . . . . I still don't know."

Wondering what it means to be physician, a mender of life, was, perhaps, Tow's major question since 1918, when her father recognized her potentials and committed himself to teach his fifth child and youngest daughter Classical Chinese Medicine at a time when women received independence, but not necessarily an education. One of the first Chinese fathers to break from convention and choose such an adventure, Dr. Chu instilled within his youngest daughter the importance of fulfilling the human being's purpose in life. Reciting from oral tradition, he would have taught:

> We are endowed at birth, both by the lineage of our ancestors and by the imprint of the heavenly bodies, to be the treasure between heaven and earth. The treasure between heaven and earth, we are to balance the influences of Yang, Heaven above, and Yin, Earth below.

By reciting this passage, Dr. Chu evoked the experience of fulfillment. By educating his daughter, he more completely realized and fulfilled his own life-purpose as a mender of life.

Dr. Chu's invocation, underscoring humankind's and physician's shared purpose, combined with his historic, life-transforming choice made fulfillment of his daughter's life-purpose a genuine possibility. Amazed in retrospect by her father's choice, which she took for granted in her youth, and amazed that she was free to accept or to refuse her father's dream for her life, Tow dramatizes through narrative dialogue her realization of her most unusual experience: an incrementally emergent mutuality between her and her father. How strange! How wonderful! Ponder the grace or the natural selection in that event. Then, mindful of our mutuality through shared purpose, she joins and converses with her reader to share her story, honor the spirit, magnify the wonder, and inspire hope. Author-reader conversations mirror Self-overheard dialogues between Tow and other persons. The aim to embody and enact genuine mutuality between all beings is a leit motif flowing and recurring beneath each event of *Strange Kindness.*

Discovery of genuine mutuality between her and her father, in what was a most significant relationship, is Tow's compositional point of departure and return—her focal point like that chosen by classical Chinese lyric poets and landscape painters. This focal point, viewed kaleidoscopically, gathers more meaning and more mystery with each new perspective. Like the focal point described by the Taoist text, *T'ai I Chin Hua Tsung, The Secret of the Golden Flower,** Tow's focus joins a still point outside of the world and ego-consciousness, a window through which she recognizes the Tao or the divine intercepting human events. Through this window, she realizes how the divine intercepted her life through the surprising choices of many people, some of whom were, at first, literally strangers. Their choices raise her wonder.

Filled with this wonder, Tow brings together in **Strange Kindness** events not only exemplifying the mutual ground of her medical art, but events intercepted by the mystery of benevolence. For instance, her anecdote, sharing how her father instructed her to heal a praying mantis, drowning in their garden pond, stresses the observed mutual healing capacities between mantis and child, physician and all creatures. These capacities exist because benevolence, the deepest thing we know, breathes through all.

We may well wonder why Dr. Chu encouraged his daughter to learn both Classical Chinese and Western, or Allopathic Medicine. Perhaps he perceived his daughter's potential to be a superior physician, a potential described by the **Huang Di Nei Jing, The Yellow Emperor's Book of Internal Medicine**:

> . . . because many changes occur in illness, the healing process must adapt to that. A superior doctor is able to gather all techniques and use them either together or separately, to flexibly adapt to a changing environment, life-style, and geography and to consider many variables in the treatment of a condition.[1]

Knowing this text and perceiving his daughter's potential, Dr. Chu perhaps selected a goal in accord with the thousand year view: the view that integrative, holistic medicine between east and west is a superior goal, one of which his daughter would be worthy.

Knowing this text, her gifted capacity to be at one with the universe, and her father's dream for her life, Tow accepted the opportunity to learn western medical arts from Episcopal missionaries in Shanghai. Her gifts and her thorough education in the holistics of Classical Chinese Medicine—the view that the liver, for example, is in a bio-psycho-dynamic-spiritual relationship with all the other bodily organs and functions, requiring physicians to regard and to treat the whole person with respect to the underlying cause of illness—all prepared her to offer a holistic and integrative approach to studying western medicine. A keen observation prepared her to study anesthesia in 1948 with the Drs. William and Charles Mayo and other staff, who had been pioneering holistic medicine in the United States since the 1920's.

With a retrospective view of Mayo's ethics and practice of holistic medicine, Martin Adson describes in his essay, *An Endangered Ethic—the Capacity for Caring,* the healing energy created by a reciprocal caregiver-patient relationship. Not unusual for four or five Mayo physicians to collaborate in the diagnosis and treatment of one patient, their practice aimed to catalyze the agent of healing within all. Physicians were to aim to embody the "kindness, evident friendly interest, acknowledgment of the patient's importance, and concern about his or her happiness," which the surgeon, James Priestly found crucial to a reciprocal, humanitarian caregiver-patient relationship.[2] To genuine kindness and care, Adson adds the operative virtues of listening, attention, presence, and dialogue. These practices flowed naturally from Tow's capacity to be at one with the universe. Her healing gift to awaken the noble heart and her attuned presence positively influenced the dynamics and vicissitudes of the surgeon-caregiver-patient relationship. These gifts and practices, her openness, flexibility and humility, disciplined by Taoist teachings, all suited her to face the unknown in each surgery and to continue to learn throughout her career as a nurse-anesthetist.

So significant, nonetheless, were Tow's early eleven years (1918–1929) of absorbing a classical Chinese education in medicine that, following almost fifty years of practice as a surgical nurse and nurse-anesthetist, she remembered at the age of eighty for her friend, Charles Liu all the meridians, acupuncture points, many herbal formulas, qigong, and the terms of practice. Tow's astonishing memory inspires the question: To what extent could she apply her early learning within western medical contexts? To what extent did the constraints and exigencies of western medicine require her to suppress her early learning?

Though we cannot definitively answer these questions, the following commentary writers offer a range of possibilities, enhancing the reader's understanding of the kind of education that Tow received, the kind of learning that she brought to her medical practice, and the kind of learning that forms a major subtext and context of her oral history.

Through words attributed to Lao Tzu, *Kindness in Words Creates Confidence*, Guangying Zhou, a research scholar, physician, and teacher of Chinese Medicine, reflects upon how Tow's living example touches our hearts to make us better people and in the process better healers.

In *Benevolence, Courage, Humility, and Keen Observation: Tow's Classical Chinese Medical Arts*, Tow's life-long friend, Charles Liu, a health educator who practices Chinese acupressure and who teaches qigong and tai chi, shares Tow's extraordinary memory of Classical Chinese Medicine and qigong. He then offers his understanding of how Tow's practice of qigong may have contributed to her practice as a nurse-anesthetist.

Lily Tsang, a teacher of Mandarin Chinese, who studied Classical Chinese Literature, reads **Strange Kindness** from Confucian and Taoist perspectives.

Stephen Rojcewicz, a psychiatrist, poetry therapist, poet and translator, reads the harmony of *kindness* and *strange*. He reads **Strange Kindness** through the lenses of holistic, western medical art and poetry therapy, finding that Tow's "life and writings provide a new synthesis, the harmony of western technological medicine with the wisdom of traditional Chinese medicine."

In *Little Bamboo: A Five-Element Study of a Life Fully Lived*, David Naimon, a naturopath and physician of Chinese Medicine, offers a reading of **Strange Kindness** through the lens of Five-Element Chinese Medicine.

In *Heart-mind Biopoetics and Tow's Moon Door*, Melissa Ann Reed, a scholar of speech-interpretation, Shakespeare dramaturge, poet, and Tow's life-long friend, shares a biopoetic understanding of Tow's healing art and the specific mending dialogue of **Strange Kindness**.

Tow's life-long friend, Vay Liang William Go, a physician, professor of medicine, and editor shares his perspective in *Mabel Cho-Shin Tow*.

Each reader and writer follows a different thread from Tow's mending dialogue. When the poet, William Stafford said that *there is a thread you follow*, he may have been referring to the thread of bliss, that thread that guides us to ripen and to fulfill our individual destinies. He may have been referring to his predecessor, E. B. White and to *Charlotte's Web* and to an author's gift of spinning a thread to save another's life, one word at a time. He may have been referring to how another's destiny may depend upon an author's one word. Each following a different thread, commentary authors reveal a range of author-reader relationships. Our hope is that their readings may inspire and enhance your own. May you be encouraged to follow the thread that guides you to ripen.

*First translated by Richard Wilhelm and a primary influence upon Carl Gustav Jung's theory of the mandala, *The Secret of the Golden Flower* was newly translated by Thomas Cleary in 1991.

1. Ni, Maoshong, trans., *The Yellow Emperor's Book of Internal Medicine.*
2. Adson, Martin A., *An Endangered Ethic—the Capacity for Caring*, presented as the first Harrison Lecture at Mayo Clinic, Rochester, Minnesota, September 28, 1994.Abridged for publication in *Mayo Clinic Proceedings*: Mayo Foundation for Medical Education and Research, 1995.

PART ONE

STRANGE KINDNESS

1

When you are young
you are good,
but when you grow up,
you choose your own nature.

Now I am old—
have not honored
my angels—
their strange kindness.
This part of the truth is
a burden to me.
How can I honor
my angels?*

Many people,
without realizing it,
carried God's message
for my life.
They would be shocked,
maybe embarrassed,
to find themselves remembered
in a story—
the story of how they guided
me in my life's way to follow
in my father's footsteps.

---

*Tow's concept of *angel* combines Taoist teaching that human beings are the treasure between heaven and earth, whose task it is to balance earthly and heavenly qi, with Jewish and Muslim teaching that angels are human beings, often strangers, whose task it is to bear divine messages.

2

In January 1948,
Dr. Ting sent me
with twenty-two hundred dollars
to a postgraduate nursing program
at St. Mary's Hospital
in Rochester, Minnesota:
I'm going to send you over there for your vacation,
because of your hard work.

My brother won't be happy.
We've not seen each other
since the war.

You'll be gone only two years.
We'll see about getting your visa
and someone to teach you English.

I couldn't say any more
about my brother.

3

So much happened
after this moment;
so much happened before.

My father,
whose Chinese name means
Fragrance of Dew,
was a medical doctor
in Hankow.*
On my birthday,
December 31, 1914,
he named me
Chu, Cho-Shin,
meaning *Little Bamboo Fragrance.*

---

*Old enough to be his youngest daughter's grandfather, Dr. Chu was a physician of Classical Chinese Medicine, which differed from post-Cultural Revolution Traditional Chinese Medicine.

You are to follow
In my footsteps,
he determined, giving
me to my mother's arms.
Make sure my Little Bamboo's
feet are not bound.
Already it was the day after my birthday,
January 1, 1915.

Had I dressed you
like your sisters,
my mother later told me,
I would have had to bind
your feet when you turned five.
All I could do
was to dress you like a boy. *

Dressed like a boy,
I literally followed
in my father's footsteps.
Invited to accompany
him on patient rounds,
I listened carefully:
My associate and I have
just opened a pharmacy
for our patients,
he would say.
To me, he would explain,
Most of our patients are poor.
Then, turning back to his patient,
he would continue,
You may receive your medicine now
and pay later when you are able.

His associate would collaborate,
Should you be able to pay a little,
pay the pharmacy first.

---

*In 1915, the Chinese Renaissance (1916-1917) had not bloomed. The double sex standard was still stressed. The majority of parents still believed that foot binding was the only way for a girl to find a good husband. By liberating his youngest daughter from old society, which restricted the education and independence of females, Dr. Chu challenged ingrained societal constraints. Cho-Shin's career began with her father's yielding choice, permitting her to cultivate the wisdom and vital energy needed for independence.

My father would conclude,
You can pay us when you are
financially comfortable.

My father, it seems,
never made a living
from his practice.*

4

Now I realize
how unusual all of his ideas were,
even his decision,
soon after I was born,
to ask friends and relatives
to give a little gift
for his precious daughter.

A gift?
This is not according
to Chinese tradition,
some objected.
Such a gift is
only for the first-born boy.

I already had a brother
twenty years older than me.

Still, we are changing,
spoke out my father's friend.
How surprised
my father must have been
to collect enough
money to make me
a pure gold locket.
Inside he had engraved
the characters *Long Life.*

*His noble family, including a grandfather, who had served as governor of Hupi, supported Dr. Chu's medical practice.

5

Since my father wanted me
to become a lady doctor,
I was the only child
among five
allowed to read
his medical books.

Even before I was old enough to read,
I was allowed to play
just outside my father's study,
where I could make dolls
and listen through the open door
to our tutor's lesson,

Lesson means:
When you are young,
you are good,
but when you grow up,
you choose your own nature.

Who can recite
from memory?
You try,
he called upon
my older cousin.

Ren zhi chu,
began my cousin,
xing ben shan
xing xiang jin
xi . . . xi . . .

He hesitated,
and then began
all over again,
Ren zhi chu
xing ben shan
xing xiang jin
xi . . . xi . . .

I laughed.

You laugh!
Can you recite for him, Cho-Shin?
our tutor invited.

Ren zhi chu
xing ben shan
xing xiang jin
xi xiang yuan*

Thank you, Cho-Shin,
responded our tutor.
You may go,
for the time being.

Ah, there you are Cho-Shin,
discovered my father.
I thought I had lost you.

Cho-Shin recited
for her cousin today
when he could not remember
his lesson.
How old is she?
wondered our tutor.

Four-and-a-half,
replied my father.

Recommend she attend
classes earlier than usual.

My punishment?
I wondered.

*As much a part of the study of medicine as it was the study of art, poetry, nature, spirituality, and culture, **The Book of Three-Word Chants** was one of the first books used for private primary school education. Rooted in the teachings of Confucius, the chants created a continuity of primary education between the Song dynasty (968-1179 C. E.) and the period marked by the establishment of the Republic of China (1911 C.E.). This Pin-Yin version offered by a teacher of Mandarin Chinese, Felix Loo, lacks the tone indicators.

6

Until fourteen-and-a-half,
I studied Confucian tradition.
Our prayer was for sky,
earth, our country's leaders,
parents, teachers and friends.

My mother was Buddhist.

Could Cho-Shin accompany me
to my temple tomorrow?
my mother asked my father one day.

She has my consent,
obliged my father.
Then, with his index finger,
he motioned me to step aside with him.
You may go with your mother,
he cautioned me,
but do not read their books.

Why?
I wondered in silence.
I could not ask then—
did not feel like arguing
with my father.
Even now, I still wonder why?

7

Always in ill health since she gave birth to me,
my mother died when I was twelve.
My two older sisters and I combed
our dead mother's hair.*
Only then, when I began
to comb her hair, could I cry.
Not quite two years before,
our grandmother died.
All I have of my grandmother
is her photograph.

---

*Liberation and education isolated Cho-Shin, not only from women of her generation, but from her older sisters, her mother, and her grandmother.

8

My father never saw his dream for me come true.
He died when I was fifteen.

My older brother,
a general manager of the Hankow-Peking Railway Station,
looked after me.
The family guardian,
he was responsible for carrying out
our father's wishes.

He wants you to be
a medical practitioner,
he repeated to me.
I must let you attend school.

After reviewing grammar school
and attending St. Joseph's Private School for Girls,
I followed my good friend, Hilda,
to the Episcopal Missionary School for Nurses.*
There, I met Mrs. Riley.

Mrs. Riley,
what does nursing mean?

A nurse is a doctor's assistant.
Depending on your level of interest,
we will place you.
Because you want to learn medicine,
we recommend that you study more English.

Because my father wants me to become a doctor,
I think I shall struggle with English.
That was my first decision.

---

*Tow's teachers, the Anglican missionaries in China, perhaps were influenced by the mysticism of Julian of Norwich, whose strong reverence for the wonders of nature taught her the essential mysteries of grace. Such an attitude would forbid disrespect to the ancient traditions and spirituality of the Chinese people. The wisdom of the Tao and of Confucianism, in harmony with the incarnational narrative of the Christian tradition, provided a modern, global consciousness and a figurative bridge, by which Tow crossed the ocean to a new continent and to new experiences in the company of new friends.

Fine, accepted Mrs. Riley.
Between your patient care, pediatrics
and practical nursing classes here,
you may go by Pedi cab to English classes
at our other Episcopal school.

I didn't want
to disappoint my father,
so I persevered
with more than a full load of courses.

One afternoon, surrounded
by my youngest patients coping
with tuberculosis,
I received some insight.
I was teaching paper folding,
when a young boy insisted,
I want to make a helicopter!

I enjoyed his enthusiasm,
which made all of us laugh.

I don't know
how to make a helicopter,
I confessed.

He ran to another love,
while the others and I returned
to our quiet concentration.
The boy soon returned, persisting,
I want to make a helicopter!

Again, all the children laughed.

I don't know
how to make a helicopter.
Do you think
that if you make a butterfly first,
you could adapt it late
 into a helicopter?

Sure!

How old are you?
I wanted to test his dexterity.

That's right, use your fingers.
One, two, three, almost four?
Good.
I think you can make
a butterfly.
First, you fold the paper
like this.

Now you need to watch me fold,
so you can follow.
That's right.
Then we fold this way.

I felt a person behind me
and looked up,
Oh, Mrs. Riley.
Could you tell me,
how long will it take me
to learn English well enough
to attend medical school?

Well, that isn't easy to say,
Mrs. Riley began.
But I will tell you
that you would make a good nurse.
See how you like children
and are gentle with them?
You always can become a doctor
after becoming a nurse.

Oh, I didn't know that.
Well, I shall decide now.
I realize that my extra English
classes take time,
time I could spend
on patient care, pediatrics,
and practical nursing classes.
I don't even have time to associate
with my classmates.
So, I choose to make
my father's dream for me
two steps.
I'll become a nurse first.

Good,
breathed Mrs. Riley.
Who knows?
You may be a better nurse
for having struggled
with English.

It never occurred
to Mrs. Riley
that I would live
most of my life
in an English-speaking country.

9

Now, come with me, Cho-Shin.
Mrs. Riley led me to her desk.
Gathered around were
two other nursing students.

I am pleased to inform you three
that you have been chosen
to enter a special nursing class
here at Episcopal Church General Hospital.
All girls who enter
this school must have
an American name.

You, she turned
to the student to my left,
you are named Mola.
Your exam was half a point
higher than Cho-Shin's.
Cho-Shin, you are named
Mabel, meaning noble,
because you come from
a noble family
and because your grandfather
was governor of your hometown province.

And you, she turned to my right,
you are named Monica.
Monica means—

Mrs. Elizabeth Riley to E.R.
Mrs. Elizabeth Riley to E.R.

We never learned what Monica means.

10

I graduated with honors as an R.N.
Forty-five classmates began with me;
about twenty-three graduated with me.
I never dreamed
I could be a surgical nurse,
I confided to Dr. Shen.
My first day in surgery, I fainted.
Remember?

I am pleased
to have chosen you
to become a surgical nurse,
responded Dr. Shen.
Please accept this silver cup engraved
with your name.

That was 1935.
After graduation, Mrs. Riley invited
me to assist her with teaching bedside care.
I taught for almost two years.
My teaching ended
when I overheard
one of my classmates, Evelyn Chin,
Cho-Shin is so proud.
A group of nurses had gathered
around Evelyn.
She's proud
because Mrs. Riley praises
her for being such a perfect
teaching assistant.
Anybody can teach.
Mrs. Riley must be partial.

Mrs. Riley,
I announced the next morning,
I dislike disharmony.
I would like to work
at Shanghai Medical School.

I hate to see you leave this way,
Mrs. Riley reluctantly consented.
Let me write your resume,
to which I shall add
my own letter of recommendation.

I had hoped to find
more suitable people
with whom to work.

Eventually Mrs. Cara,
superintendent of Shanghai Medical School
and an American missionary,
shared with me Mrs. Riley's letter:
Because Cho-Shin is so good,
and because her work has contributed
so much to our nursing school,
I request that she be allowed to return
after a year with Shanghai Medical School.

That was 1937.
I never returned
to Episcopal General.

11

In 1938,
after Japanese War began,
many of our patients
were Japanese soldiers.
They would kick their nurses.

Mrs. Cara, I proposed,
I wonder if I could take off
two months to work
in Chinese refugee camp?
They need nurses, too.
I am thinking it is
my duty to care
for my own people.

Yes, I think we can arrange
that, Mrs. Cara accepted.
You may use Shanghai Medical School's
public health uniform and medical bags.

The camp was a long warehouse filled
with more than a thousand refugees.
All had to lie on straw mattresses
on the floor.

Not everyone has a mattress,
I expressed my pain to Mrs. Cara,
whose face froze in shock.

I don't think my work benefits
 them much.   All I can do
 is to feed them rice soup and water
and wash their faces.

I saw my own sadness reflected
through Mrs. Cara's face.

Every evening,
when I return home,
I soak
my lice-filled
uniform
in Lysol solution
and wash
my lice-filled
hair.

12

About six months later
Dr. Ting asked Dr. Jen
from Shanghai Medical School
to work part-time with him
at his private hospital.

I'm nearly retired, Dr. Ting.
I don't have to work,
reasoned Dr. Jen.
If you want me to be associated
with your practice,
you'd best invite Chu Cho-Shin
to work with you, too.
She's been my surgical nurse
for about three years.

Through Mrs. Cara
and the Chinese refugee camp supervisor,
Dr. Ting finally found me:
How would you like to schedule
and supervise all our surgeries?
Dr. Ting telephoned to ask.

I don't know,
I honestly replied.
How many doctors are associated
with your practice?

At present, sixteen.
Dr. Jen just joined us.
We perform six to eight surgeries a day
with sometimes an emergency surgery between.
You always would be on call.
It is perhaps too much responsibility
for someone your age.

If Dr. Jen is joining your practice,
it must be good.
He is retired.
He doesn't have to work.
I accept your offer.
Thank you.

When I accepted to work with Dr. Ting,
I could not, of course, foresee my life.
Now I realize
how I would not have today
had it not been
for Dr. Jen and Dr. Ting.

And my white cat, Kate May!

13

Kate May was born in May.
An American missionary gave her to me.

Cho-Shin,
Japanese authorities are sending
me to a concentration camp.
Would you keep Kate May?

I couldn't speak.

She chose you
from among all my friends.
Remember?
When you visited me,
she rushed out of hiding
and wrapped herself around your legs
in an embrace of friendship
she never extended
to others.

Okay,
I accepted Kate May.
I will care for her,
and I hope
I will see you again.

I remember the brush
of Kate May's long tail,
especially noticeable
when she tried to catch birds.
The long brush of her white
Persian tail extended
about me like fine tentacles,
like a sea anemone.

During blackouts
and bombings,
I would gather my three
family photo albums,
place Kate May on top,
and off we'd run
to the bomb shelter.

We didn't have far to run.
A bomb shelter waited
just outside Dr. Ting's private hospital.
Safe underground, I would wonder,
Kate May, why is it
you never try to escape?

Kate May and I were inseparable.

14

At this time, I met Dr. Yang,
an avid photographer like me.
We both spent nearly all
our spare time taking photographs.

All your photos?
Dr. Yang asked me one time
as the siren blew,
and we left the bomb shelter.

All I have of my family and friends.

*My family and friends come to mind
in the bomb shelter, too.*

*All the people I carry
in my heart rush through me
like the many names written
on my Great Grandfather's umbrella.*

An umbrella full of names?

*Yes, the umbrella was signed
by all the people of Hupi and given
to my Great Grandfather when he retired
as governor of their province.
The umbrella holds a special place
in our family house of memory.*

Many years have passed
since the bomb shelter.
Many angels have given me today.
Perhaps they would be honored
if I wrote their names
on a special memory umbrella
like the one given to my Great Grandfather.

15

When the bombings ceased,
Dr. Ting's private hospital stood intact.
It was 1944.

Most of our patients were Chinese-American,
some were Russian,
all were very poor.
Russian peasants, carrying
many blankets on their backs,
were a familiar sight.
They crossed
our border to sell
blankets to pay
for their medical care.
Even so, most patients
could not pay
for their rooms.

*I work
more than ever,*
reflected Dr. Yang,
*share my two-course meals
of soup with rice and beans,
imagine the other two courses,
and keep dreaming
I have to run
 to the bomb shelter.*

*Life is now difficult
for everyone in China,*
I responded,
*yet you and I are free
to be honorable people.
We speak our heart-truth,
are not afraid of poverty.*

I think we take our freedom for granted,
warned Dr. Yang.

Between 1946 and 1947,
when Dr. Ting visited
all the well-known hospitals
and clinics in the United States,
our loyalties and freedom were tested.

One afternoon,
an orderly rushed
into my office,

Miss Chu,
will you please come
to our meeting
tonight at eight?
I couldn't make
the others understand
my feeling.
I think they would listen to you.

Do you know their complaint?

They want to eat as normal.
They suspect some of us receive
preferential treatment.

I dislike disharmony.
How many 'others' are there?

Nineteen.

Nineteen of Dr. Ting's
twenty-one employees.
Nineteen had forgotten Dr. Ting,
who cared so much
about giving his patients
the best possible
medical care.

A room full of strikers spoke out
to me all at once.

I cannot understand everyone at once,
I addressed them.
One or two of you speak at a time.

We eat only two dishes,
complained one.

Dr. Ting is off to enjoy himself,
accused another.

While we have to suffer alone,
concluded the first.

While Dr. Ting eats well in the U.S.
continued the second,
we wonder who else eats
better than we do at home?

You eat only two dishes,
I began.
We staff eat the same two dishes.
I am sure Dr. Ting would be eating
the same way we do.
He is one of us.
You can see that everyone has trouble.
Patients cannot always pay for their rooms.
It isn't just you or us.
This isn't Dr. Ting's doing.
It is our country that is in trouble.
Don't you think we all
would like to have peace?
No more war?
Because of war,
everyone has difficulty.
Let's remember our benefits
and Dr. Ting's care.

I turned to the first striker,
Your wife just had a baby in this hospital.
she received complete care—
didn't pay a penny.

All became quiet.

Thank you, Miss Chu,
bowed the orderly.
You may go now,
if you wish.

During the nine years
between 1939 and 1948
that I worked for Dr. Ting,
I was, of course, too immersed
in my work to regard him an angel.
Besides he was Buddhist.
He never would have thought
of himself as an angel.

16

Why do you wish me
to study at Mayo?
I questioned Dr. Ting
that fateful day
in January 1948.

I especially like the Mayo Clinic.
Doctors work together,
make mutual decisions
with their patients.
I see how this practice contributes
to giving the best medical care.

What do you suggest
I study there?

Either physical medicine
or anesthesia.
I told Sister Mary Brigh
that you are responsible,
always please your patients,
even deliver babies
when doctors are unavailable.
Sister Mary Brigh said,
"Send her right away."

Dr. Ting is surely one
of my angels.
Had it not been for Dr. Ting,
I would have stayed in China.
Had I stayed in China,
I would have had to taste
the spirit of freedom leaving my home.
Not that I escaped suffering.*

17

Your photograph, Miss Chu,
presented Dr. Yang
just before I left China.

*Recognizing that all could have happened otherwise, Tow suffers with her people, as well as she suffers from being separated from them.

He had photographed me sitting
beside the lake, where I often sat,
talking to the moon.
Later, I wrote a poem
about our conversation
to honor the spirit of freedom between us.

> Moonlight shines
> through tree branches
> into my heart.
>
> I don't like you
> when you try to learn
> my secret.
>
> I love you
> when you let me tell you
> what I want to tell you.

Had I stayed in China,
I would not have been permitted
to speak my heart-mind—
to tell you what I am free to tell you.
In China, my choices
would have been forced.
I could not have been true
to my father's dream,
could not have followed
in my father's footsteps.
Still, I was not spared suffering.

Hardest to leave
was Kate May.
I still remember
what a good hunter she was.

What? Another mouse!
I always praised her.
Too bad you eat only milk and beef,
both scarce.
We must find a way to thank our kind-hearted cook.
Each time she makes soup,
she gives up her own portion
so you may enjoy
a half cup of beef and a pint of milk
every day.

Kate May was
(and still is)
my connection with China.

Forty people,
all close friends and co-workers,
gathered in the ship-yard
to see me off.

Goody-bye, Dr. Yang,
I began the long litany of farewells.
Please accept
one of my photos called,
"If you want to see further,
you have to climb higher."

Oh, thank you.
Good-bye, Miss Chu,
and good luck!

Neighbors came,
even the parents of a boy
whom I delivered,
and another of my angels,
Dr. Jen.

Good-bye, Dr. Jen.
I shall miss you.

Had it not been for Dr. Jen,
Dr. Ting and I would not have met.

After waving more good-byes,
I entered the ship's cabin.

Li Sung Pe!
Are you traveling, too?
I asked the smiling gentleman,
who was just like a good uncle,
seated at one of the tables.

Wish I could,
he responded.
I just boarded
to surprise you.

All those farewells
would have left me feeling empty
had it not been for Dr. Ting's parting words,
You look as if you have lost
something—someone.
He read my emptiness.

Kate May.
All I can think of is
my white Persian cat
with her one green eye
and one blue.

She'll be waiting for you.
Now, if you need more money,
just let me know.

I doubted needing more money.
Still wonder why Dr. Ting gave me so much.
Twenty-two hundred dollars!
His thought and his kindness stayed
in my heart, stayed
like the memory
of Katie May.

18

When the S. S. President Cleveland
finally began her maiden trip
from China to America,
I felt as if I were going to spend
only two weeks in another Chinese city.

I also felt seasick for the first time in my life.

Paul Natividad,
the ship steward, tended
to those of us who became seasick,
This time, I brought you Chinese food cooked
just right for you, Miss Chu.

I can't.
Not even Chinese food.

So he brought me desserts
the way that Kate May used to bring me birds and mice,
How about pudding and ice cream from first class trays?
Nobody's touched it.

Nobody?
I accepted the tray.
Nobody's touched it,
I can still hear him say.

More ice cream for you, Miss Chu?
Nobody's touched it.

One time, when I accepted
Paul's ice cream tray,
He confided,
My father died,
and my mother is Chinese.
They would be so happy to know
I can give you some nourishment.

His words touch a memory.
I am back home in Hankow.
My father is dredging
the pond in our backyard.
I am perched on the edge
opposite him,
Father, come!
What is this insect?
I've never seen it before.
Look, it's drowning.
It's all wet and cannot fly.

Oh, he's good for you
He's a praying mantis.
Wait here, while I fetch
you a long stick.

Here,
returned my father,
a little out of breath.
Gently hold out this stick for the mantis.
Soon, he'll begin to pray.

I was a nine-year-old then,
full of pretty good insights.
This was also the first time
I challenged my father,
How do you know?

When he feels better,
he will show you himself.
He's all wet now.
He can't pray.
Here, let's turn him around.
There now.
Hold this stick longer
until he recovers.

But he looks dead.

Just wait.
I think he is going to live.

My father returned
to dredge the pond.
I settled down to wait
for the mantis to recover
and pray.

Ah look, father,
he is trying to spread his wings.
*He **is** going to live.*

Yes.
Yes, I think he is okay now.
Let's place him on your finger.

Where?
Is he going to bite me?

No, he won't bite.
We'll put him on your thumb
where he can remove that wart.

Oh, he smells something.
He's eating my wart,
and I don't feel any pain.
Look, he's eating roots and all.

You see?
Now observe.
Two little legs are together.
That's praying.
You watch the mantis pray,
while I check your finger.
Hmmmm, looks good.
Two healings, the mantis's and yours.
That's good. That's good.
Now place him on this towel.
That's right.
When he becomes stronger,
he may fly away.

Okay, I'll watch the mantis.
You go back, dredge the pond.
We saved your life, little mantis,
you removed my wart,
and then you said your prayers.
That's good. That's good.
Oh father,
you want to come?
He's flying away now.

Wonderful.

Why?

We are not supposed to keep them.
We are to let them go free.

Good-bye!
We saved your life;
you removed my wart.

Like my father,
Paul Natividad was
a genuinely kind person.
He saved my life
the way my father saved
the praying mantis's life.
Paul is another person,
who gave me today.
He is another angel to keep
on my umbrella.

19

February sixth,
nineteen forty eight,
we arrived in San Francisco.
One of our landing party,
Bishop Stephen Tsang
introduced me to Father Reese,
who frugally settled me
into the Stuart Hotel.
Here we are, my little lamb.

Fireworks exploded.
I questioned the steward,
Why all the noise?

Aren't you Chinese?
It's Chinese New Year.
Don't you celebrate that at home?

Not with fireworks,
not after Japanese War.

The steward's assumptions annoyed
me, and the fireworks reminded
me of bomb shelter days.
The ten days I stayed in San Francisco
would have been unbearable
without Father Reese.

20

Another angel,
Father Reese kept me under his wing.
I can still hear him,
Here we are now.
This is Fisherman's Wharf.
Mabel . . . Mabel?
(I found it difficult at first
to respond to my American name.)
Mabel, you sit here by the window.
That's right.
Now you can see the harbor.
Ann, you sit next to Mabel over there.
I'll sit by her here.

He held a chair for Mrs. Reese
adjacent himself.
Mabel is our little lamb now.

What do you think of Chinatown, Mabel?
queried Mrs. Reese.

*Makes me feel unreal
to be in such a place
in a foreign country.*

May I take your orders now?
interrupted a waiter.

Seated at Fisherman's Wharf,
I could smell all my favorite food:
crab, shrimp—

*Yes, bring Mabel a steak,
medium rare,*
ordered Father Reese.

Oh, you order for me?
I wondered as the waiter repeated
the order in his book,
Steak, medium rare.

To order for me
was a generosity
to which I was unaccustomed.

How could Father Reese have known
that, since the cow is blessed
in China, I am forbidden
to eat beef?

*Mabel, you haven't touched
your food,* noticed
the Reese's daughter, Ann.

*Since I get off boat,
I don't feel like to eat much.
In China, we show guests about our cities,
but we don't spend money on them.*

We wouldn't find a place
for them to stay,
unless of course they asked us.
Not otherwise.
I haven't asked for anything.
Seems like we've been friends
for a long time.

You are most welcome, Mabel,
accepted Mrs. Reese.

At the time, I couldn't explain
about the cow,
about how, being the one to plow
the rice, the cow is blessed.
My English wasn't good enough.
Now I see it was best not to explain.
It was best to be gracious.
Oh, I cannot forget Father Reese.

21

I still remember
the telephone ringing
and Father Reese answering,
Hello . . .
Yes, Mrs. Raven . . .
Ah, yes, Dr. T ing asked you to call for Mabel.
Well, you don't have to worry about Mabel.
. . . Yes, yes, I'm showing her San Francisco.
. . . We've been to Fisherman's Wharf.
. . . Yes, yes, we've been to Chinatown.
. . . Oh, we've already taken the Harborview Drive.
. . . Yes, yes, we've seen the mansions.
. . . Yes, yes, you may have her phone number
and her address at the Stuart Hotel.
You can reach her any time.
Yes. Good-bye now, Mrs. Raven.

Ann and Mrs. Reese and I laughed
at the overheard conversation.
He's such a mother hen, isn't he?
enjoyed Mrs. Reese.

Oh, I nearly forgot!
I remembered.
I've packed some gifts
for my new friends in America.
They are in my trunk,
full of medicine.
I ran to my steamer trunk
by Reese's front door
and rummaged through
to the gifts at the bottom.

You brought medicine from China?
Ann was astonished.

Dr. Ting insisted.
Someone on the ship may need care.
Let's see, Ann, would you like
a glass dog and a glass bird?

Oh, they are lovely.

And please accept my own Chinese dress.

How beautiful, breathed Mrs. Reese.
White satin with pink flowers.

I shall keep this dress 'til I die,
accepted Ann.

Now let me take your pictures,
Father Reese insisted.

The ease with which Father Reese managed
my life, giving poor Mrs. Raven
all of about three visits with me,
was part of his natural affection.
Couldn't forget Father Reese.

22

Soon it was time for me to buy
a train ticket to Rochester.

All are boarding now,
announced Father Reese.

Here's your ferryboat ticket,
and here's your train ticket,
both at a special student rate.

Oh, thank you,
I fished for coins in my purse.
Here.
Is that right amount?

I always think you know what to do,
yet you really don't,
realized Father Reese,
sad for the first time.
Can I give you a hug?

I don't know.
What is a hug?

Father Reese gave me
my first hug,
There.
I pray for you.
You are going to be all right.

If everyone in this country is
like Father Reese, I dreamed,
then I really have come to heaven.

When our ferry launched out,
however, I became worried.
I wondered how I would know
where to go,
which train to board.

Then an idea occurred to me.
I opened my suitcase,
found a piece of paper,
and printed in large letters,
WHERE ARE YOU GOING?
Then I pinned the sign
to the front of my dress.

Oh, where are you going, dear?
offered a stout, middle-aged lady.

Rochester, Minnesota.
Can I go with you?
I've never taken this train.
This is my first time in this country.

Of course you may go with me,
accepted the kind lady.
You'll be on the right train,
Don't worry; I take the same train to St. Cloud.
You get off just before me.

Oh, thank you!
Could you help me, too?
Let me learn what to do?

From now on, we'll sit, walk and dine together.

Though I cannot recall
this lady's name,
she is another angel.
I shall remember her
the St. Cloud Lady.

Can I beg you to do something for me?
the St. Cloud lady spoke up
while we unpacked
by our sleeping berths.

Sure.

Just look at me.
I'm way too large to climb
up on the upper berth.
Would you take it?

It is ok.
Fine with me.
It was as if God had chosen
us to be perfect friends.

So why are you going to Rochester?
wondered my new friend.

To study anesthesia.

I told her the whole story.
How Dr. Ting had ordered,
I'm going to send you over there
for your vacation,
because of your hard work.
How I had resisted,
My brother won't be happy.
We've not seen each other
since the war.
How Dr. Ting promised,
You'll be gone only two years.
We'll see about getting your visa
and someone to teach you English.
How I couldn't say any more
about my brother.

How sad, dear,
reflected my new friend.

I'll be gone only two years,
I comforted her.

Two years.
My vacation!
Sounds funny to me now.

It's February eighteenth already,
the St. Cloud lady announced,
repacking her suitcase.
Time for us to part company.
You won't have time for lunch today, dear.
We'll arrive in Rochester between
ten and eleven a.m.
So we'll share a good breakfast, ok?

Ok.

I had no trouble from San Francisco to Rochester
because of this genuinely considerate person.

It's quarter to ten, dear.
Let's get your luggage together.
After we arrive in Rochester,
you let me call a cab for you.
I know I'll think about you many times.

I'm beginning to miss you already.
I hope your work in surgery goes well.
Hope you can come to visit me in St. Cloud.

23

I was thirty-four years old
when I arrived at St. Mary's.
I see now from my photo
that I looked sixteen.
Many an undiscerning person,
like Dr. Sam, treated
me almost like a youngster.
You're a liar, he teased.
How can you be thirty-four?
You don't even look twenty!

Yes, that's true,
agreed Sister Mary Brigh,
but she has supervised
surgeries for sixteen doctors
and delivered babies.

That's true,
I smiled.
Sister Mary Brigh was different.
She was respectful.

Dr. Ting also said
you speak fluent English.

Not too much,
I admitted.
We didn't much need
to speak English in Shanghai.

But you were with American missionaries,
began Sr. Mary Brigh in disbelief.

Yes, I acknowledged,
but they wanted to learn Chinese.

We laughed.

Do I have to have social security?
The question suddenly popped into my head.
A lady on the train told me
I would need it.

No, you don't have to apply for it now.
You are a student.
There is one thing you need, though.
Dr. Ting tells me
your American name is Mabel.
I think you should have a nickname.

Nickname?

Yes, a name of endearment.
What we give to someone
when we especially like them.

I nodded with understanding.

We'll call you Chu-Chu,
determined Sr. Mary Brigh.
Already my angel,
she had me under her wing.
It never occurred to me then
I would never again see my brother.

24

Chu-Chu!
Dr. Sam recognized me
when we met in the subway one morning.

Don't you remember me, Chu-Chu?
I'm Dr. Sam.
You look lost.

I am to study
with Sr. Remanda,
the surgical supervisor,
I replied.
I don't like to be late my first day.

Just take this subway straight ahead,
directed Dr. Sam.

It connects Marian Hall,
where you are now,
with the hospital.

Thank you.

I still got lost in the subway.
God, I prayed,
I don't know how much I can do,
or how long I can do,
or how fast I can learn.
I only remember the Bible story
about people who turned against you,
people who built a Tower of Babel.
I remember how you became so angry
you made everyone speak a different language.
If you can make people speak different languages,
will you give me wisdom to use English?

Praying gave me a little hope.

25

The first person
with whom I could converse at length
was my Marian Hall roommate,
Mary Angelbeck.

Oh, you must be hungry!
Mary exclaimed as we selected
food from the hospital cafeteria.

What do you mean?
I wondered.

You chose all main dishes—
three entrees.

I thought we were to have
five dishes for the main meal.

That is a formal dinner.
Since the end of the war,
we stopped serving five courses.

Still confused,
I looked down at my tray.

Look, Mary tried to explain,
you don't have as much as one serving,
but all variety.
You spend more money than you need to.

I still don't understand.
What are you saying?

Choose one main dish,
then a vegetable, a salad, and bread.
How much do you pay?

Four dollars, twenty-five cents.

Quick, come with me,
Mary invited.
I'll show you.

Quickly we passed behind table
after table as Mary showed me
everyone's plate.
After the lesson, Mary paused,
What did you see?

Just as you say.
I understand.
Thank you.

Now, you didn't pour milk.
Just water.
You need milk.
If you choose five entrees,
the cost is between thirty-five
and forty dollars a month.
This other way,
your cost is only
twenty-five or thirty a month.
You'll have money to buy milk.

Because of Mary Angelbeck's advice,
I learned to save money.
I see God's love in her guidance.

Maybe it is not for me to tell you,
began Mary,
yet it is right for you to know.
If I hadn't told you,
who else would?
I like you, Chu-Chu,
not just because you gave me a gift,
but because we are going to be good friends,
confided my friend and angel, Mary Angelbeck.

26

As postgraduates,
we worked during the day
and attended class in the evening.
Only weekends offered free time,
time to make pictures.

Now let's photograph you, Chu-Chu,
Mary Angelbeck suggested one afternoon.
You look like a dream in that dress.

I like butterflies,
admired my new friend,
Dr. Janet Wong.

I love butterflies,
especially when they fly,
I elaborated.

Stand right by that pink almond bush,
directed Dr. Chen, Janet's husband.
That's right,
he focused his camera.

Once, when I was a child,
I began my story,
My first cat was
in my father's garden with me.
A butterfly alighted on his ear.
When my father charged
with a fly-swatter,
the cat ran away.
You didn't educate your cat well,
scolded my father.

He doesn't know I love you—
wouldn't kill him,
much less the butterfly.

When I smiled,
Dr. Chen snapped the photo.

Moments in my father's garden return to me
in a flash.
In a flash,
I am there, flown home
like a butterfly.
In another flash,
I am back at St. Mary's,
back to coursework,
back to learning English,
one of ten postgraduates,
each of us a different nationality.

By mid-October,
all ten postgraduates were photographed
for the **Rochester Post Bulletin.**

Then Dr. Tao's letter arrived:
Dear Cho-Shin,
I heard you are here in the U.S.
at St. Mary's Hospital.
I'm so sorry I didn't let you know
where I went when I left China.
I am practicing in Pennsylvania.

Please know that if you are here
without an immigrant visa,
you must not accept pay.
If you accept pay,
you will be deported.
Sincerely,
Dr. Chang Tse Tao

Immediately my memory flashed back
to a conversation with Sr. Mary Brigh,
Chu-Chu,
your country is going to be in trouble.
The Communist War began this past July.
Maybe Dr. Ting cannot send you money so easily now.

Since we want you to remain in our program,
we will pay you.

Immediately I showed Sr. Mary Brigh
Dr. Tao's letter.

Don't worry, Chu-Chu,
Sr. Mary Brigh assured me.
We shall give you fellowship pay.

That was Friday.
Friday night,
our photographs appeared
in the **Post Bulletin**
Monday morning,
Mr. Hansen of immigration appeared
in Sr. Mary Brigh's office.

I checked out everyone
in your postgraduate program,
Sr. Mary Brigh.
All have support
from their home hospital
except Miss Chu.
She is on your payroll.
Miss Chu, did you tell Sr. Mary Brigh
that you cannot accept pay?

Yes.

Sr. Mary Brigh,
did Miss Chu tell you
she cannot accept pay
without severe consequences?

Sr. Mary Brigh bowed
her head and nodded,
Yes.

That is all for now,
Mr. Hansen dismissed us
and left.

I'm so sorry, Chu-Chu,
Sr. Mary Brigh apologized.

I went on retreat,
forgot to change your name
to fellowship.
When immigration called,
I could not explain.
I hope you can stay.
If not,
I hope you can come back.

Shocked,
I could only be glad
that writing to Dr. Ting
was an impossibility.
Word soon came
that I had to leave Rochester
by the end of January 1949.
Mary Angelbeck found me packing.

Some think
that Dr. Mayo and
Mr. Graham will write
to congressmen on your behalf,
she tried to comfort me.

A messenger brought
the response,
A letter for you,
Miss Chu.
Hope it's good news.

Dear Miss Chu,
I would love you to be here.
I don't know immigration, though.
If I spent time with them,
I could not practice medicine,
and medicine is my life's work.
My heart is crossed for you.
I would love to fight for you,
but I just cannot.
Sincerely,
Dr. Charles Mayo

I had worked
a month and a half
in surgery

with Dr. Mayo
and Dr. Walters
and then five months
with Dr. Waugh,
a fellow
with the Mayo group.
So when Dr. Waugh's wife,
Amy,
invited me
to their annual
Christmas Eve party,
she already knew
I had to leave Rochester
in January.

Oh, Mabel,
Amy greeted me at her front door,
I'm so glad you came.
Won't you come in, dear?

Slowly,
I entered
a warm,
magical room.
Let's have a picture,
demanded Dr. Sam.
Smile.
Good!
He snapped our picture,
then looked for another shot.

May I call you Chu-Chu?
wondered Amy.

Please,
I accepted.

My husband tells me
how much he enjoys working with you.
There's Dr. Waugh with Dr. Walters
over there with that group.

Mmmmmm,
I breathed in the aroma.
I like pine fragrance.

Well, here are the decorations,
all from years past,
reminisced Amy.
Choose what you'd like to hang,
she invited me to trim the tree.

Oh, I like the silver tinsel,
I admired.

Good.
You tinsel the tree.
Oh, and here's Dr. Sam.

May I join you?
I like tinsel, too,
chimed in Dr. Sam.

Ok, laughed Amy.
You tinsel one side, Sam,
and Chu-Chu may tinsel the other.
I'll welcome you with some piano music.
My uncle taught me this song.
If you understand, Chu-Chu,
then I've remembered it right.
If not, then I've forgotten.

She played *Jesus Loves Me,*
singing the words in Chinese.
I listened at first
and then joined her.

You have a good memory,
I complimented Amy.

My uncle taught me the words.
He was a missionary to China.

Our friendship started that way.
Never ended.
So, on Christmas Eve, 1948,
God gave me another angel.

Well, everyone,
let's admire the tree,
announced Amy.

Chu-Chu, you come, too.
Let's see how your partner's side looks.
Oh, I think he tossed the tinsel.
Now, let's inspect your side.
Ah, yes, hung like graceful icicles.
Which of the sides do you like best, Chu-Chu?

I think each side is ok,
if it is enjoyed in its own way,
I reflected, offering
the natural Chinese way of receiving
art and humankind's creative expression.

I think you are smart,
applauded Amy.

27

When January 29th arrived,
Amy cleaned out
the trunk of her car
to carry my luggage,
bundled her two children
(home from school for lunch)
into the backseat,
and accompanied me
to the railway station.

Now, as I was saying, Chu-Chu,
I always ask myself,
Amy, how is it you have today?

With understanding,
we kissed each other good-bye.

You know, Chu-Chu,
I think we will
see each other again.

Because of Amy,
I still had hope.

As the train departed,
Amy and her children and I waved
our good-byes.

Then I re-read Dr. Waugh's letter:
Dear Chu-Chu,
We pray for you.
We would love for you to stay,
but we must attend our patients.
We cannot do that and work
with politicians, too.
Sincerely,
Dr. Waugh

Like Dr. Mayo,
Dr. Waugh was being honest.
My thoughts turned to reports
of my patients' affections for me.
You know, Sr. Mary Brigh,
Sr. Remanda shared,
our patients favor Chu-Chu.
They always ask for her.
"When is Chu-Chu coming back"
"Is Chu-Chu on duty today?"
"We feel better when Chu-Chu changes our dressings.
We'll wait for her."

Understandably so,
appreciated Sr. Mary Brigh.
Chu-Chu never uses our surgical tape.
"Pulls patients' skin off," she says.
She always ties dressings in place
the way they are tied in China.

Their voices faded.
I felt lost.
I was supposed to become
an anesthetist,
study anesthesia for two years.

God,
I prayed,
If you don't think
I should be an anesthetist,
then just give me peace.

Though peace came to me,
I was never satisfied.

What could I do to change
my circumstance?
How could I start over again?
I couldn't practice
as a nurse in the U.S.
My R.N. had been received in China.
Couldn't be applied here.

The train accelerated,
and we were well
on our way to New York.

Though my study of anesthesia
would resume in 1952,
that January 1949,
I never dreamed it possible.
I felt as though my dream
had just been snatched
away from me.

Then I remembered
Amy Waugh's question,
How is it that you have today?

My thoughts turned
to a strange conversation
with Mr. Anderson,
the railway clerk in Rochester.
Let's see,
he advised, checking schedules,
*You'd like to see your schoolmate in New York,
and then Father Reese in San Francisco.*
(At one time, Father Reese had promised
to give me a job for room and board.)

Oh, but wait,
I dreamed a little.

*Before I go to San Francisco,
I would like to see Washington, D.C.*

*I'm not going to give you
a ticket to Washington, D.C.,*
replied Mr. Anderson.
You buy a round-trip ticket

from New York to D.C.
It's only twelve dollars that way.
From Rochester to New York is ok.
Come back to Chicago first, though,
and then continue from Chicago to San Francisco.
This way I can save you fifty-six dollars.

How strange these directions sounded to me then.
Now they sound prophetic.
How could the railway clerk have known
I would meet my future husband in New York
and wind up living in Chicago?
He couldn't have known.

Mr. Anderson must be one of my angels.

28

In New York,
I met my schoolmate,
Pang Sen Dutsen,
meaning *person of high character.*

Late one afternoon,
Dutsen invited me to a curio shop
filled with Chinese artifacts,
Come, Cho-Shin,
see the wonderful jade
kept under glass.
Just then, the curio shop owner looked up
to recognize his cousin walking in,
Frank, what a surprise to see you!

I'm here to attend
Chinese Family Association Convention.
Thought I'd come see some of my family,
smiled Frank.

I knew you were coming to this convention.
You are the chairman.
I never dreamed
you would come to see me.
Come, meet my visitors.
Pang Sen Dutsen and Chu Cho-Shin,
this is my cousin, Frank Tow.

We bowed to one another.
Then Frank turned away to speak
privately with his cousin.
Dutsen and I continued to browse.

Dutsen! Dutsen!
beckoned Frank's cousin.

Excuse me a moment, Cho-Shin,
requested Dutsen,
walking to Frank's cousin's side.

*Dutsen, my cousin would like to take
Cho-Shin out for dinner.*

I watched Dutsen nod
and cross to me,
*Cho-Shin, Frank Tow's cousin tells me
Frank would like to take you out for dinner.*

No!
I was adamant.
*I don't want to make friends.
I don't know where I'm going to be.
First, I have to see Father Reese.*

Dutsen nodded her understanding,
and then re-crossed to Frank's cousin,
*"No," she says.
She doesn't know
where she is going to be.
First, she has to see Father Reese.*

They exchanged perplexed glances.

Cho-Shin, come with me,
beckoned Frank's cousin.
He guided me to a back room and lectured,
*You are in the United States now.
Don't be this way.
My cousin is a good man from Chicago.
He's chairing the Chinese Family Association Convention
here in New York.
I knew he was attending this convention.
I didn't know he would come to see me.*

If he takes you out for dinner, it's ok.
You don't have to feel you owe him anything.
He wants good company,
so he asked you.

We returned to the front of the curio shop.
Dutsen immediately gathered me to her side,
He's a good man, Cho-Shin.
You go.
I'll wait for you at home.

At the time, I didn't even know
how to order food,
and since I spoke only Mandarin
and Frank spoke only Cantonese,
we could communicate
only in broken English.

Whatever you like to order, go ahead,
encouraged Frank.

I don't know how to order.
Whatever you like to order, order for me, too,
I deferred.

I like fish.
Do you like fish?

Yes,
I brightened.

Then, we'll order pan fried fish and salad.
Tell me,
why did you leave China?

To study anesthesia at Mayo.

I told Frank the whole story,
beginning with Dr. Ting's gift,
I'm going to send you over there as your vacation
because of your hard work.

My brother won't be happy.
We've not seen each other since the war.

You'll be gone only two years.
We'll see about getting your visa
and someone to teach you English.

I couldn't say any more
about my brother, I reflected.
Now—

Now you are here in New York
about to enjoy pan fried fish and salad.
Tell me, if you want to,
why did you leave Mayo?

By mistake.

Mistake?

By mistake,
my name was on payroll
instead of fellowship.

Then you were almost deported?

Almost.
Now I see my blessing.
Thank you.

We'll go somewhere else now,
Frank abruptly stood up.

My friend—
I began to decline the invitation,
but Frank was not listening.
He left a tip on the table and walked
straightaway to the cashier.

Thank you, sir.
Have a good evening,
wished the cashier
as Frank walked out
to hail a taxi.

I don't think I should—
I declined,
but Frank was focused elsewhere.

Taxi!

Before I could say *no,*
we were taxied to Radio City Music Hall,
then to a Laurel and Hardy double feature,
then—*I think I'd like to go somewhere else,*
announced Frank like a youngster.

My friend is waiting for me,
I firmly explained.
It's already midnight.
I don't think I should stay out too late.

You are good,
if you think about your friend,
complimented Frank.

Taxi!
We'll take you home.
Taxi!

I marveled at the speed
of New York taxi drivers.
Before I could think
or say *thank you,*
Frank spoke up,
I never knew I'd meet you today.

My building is two blocks away,
I directed the taxi driver.

I had a wonderful time,
Frank continued.

Right here is fine,
I assured the driver.

I wish we had time to talk more,
Frank motioned the driver to wait
and helped me out of the taxi.
Since we can't talk,
let me ask.
Would you marry me?

I became rigid.

Without saying a word,
I quickly walked away.

Is there anything wrong?
Dutsen wondered
as I flew past her
on the way to my room.
You look so different.

No, nothing is wrong.

Well, here,
Dutsen offered,
have some cookies and milk.

29

At eight o'clock the next morning,
Dutsen was making oatmeal,
and I was peeling an orange
when the telephone rang.
Dutsen answered,
Hello.
. . . Yes, Frank.
Just a moment.

I shook my hand, indicating
I didn't want to talk.

She's busy now.
Can you call later?

Ten o'clock,
the telephone rang again.
I was embroidering.
Dutsen answered,
Hello.
. . . Yes, Frank.
Just a moment.

Again I shook my hand, indicating
I didn't want to talk.

Hadn't you better thank him for last night?
cajoled Dutsen.

You never said a word.
However you feel,
you cannot forget your manners.

You lecture me
as though I were a youngster.

I picked up the receiver,
and just the way I had always apologized
to my older sister at my father's request,
I apologized to Frank,
I'm sorry
I didn't thank you
for the good time.

That's ok.
I'm at the airport.
Just bought something
for our restaurant.
Since my plane is delayed two hours,
would you take a cab to the airport
so we can talk?
I can tell you how I feel.
I'll send you home by cab.

No, I'm not going,
I hung up.

Mabel!
Dutsen was astonished.

I don't know
what kind of person he is,
I defended.
His past is unknown to me.
I don't think I should mingle with him.

So, I didn't go to meet Frank at the airport,
didn't tell him why.
I was so immersed
in our Chinese custom
that I didn't realize
how silly I was being
in the new circumstance.

In China,
I reiterated to Dutsen,
women don't go out
with strangers.
Marriages in China are matched
by our fathers.
My father wished me to follow
in his footsteps,
become a doctor.
He never said anything about marriage.
Even if he had,
a couple's families
are supposed to attend
a tea house together.
If they converse well,
then they return to the tea house
for more conversation.

Did you and Frank converse well?
wondered Dutsen.

A couple must shake hands with their parents,
before they can talk.
I continued my litany of tradition.
These customs were so a part of me
that any kind of relationship with Frank
seemed to be not only absurd,
but highly impossible.

The telephone rang.
Yes, this is Mabel.

This is Frank.
I'm in Chicago now.
Have to talk to you.
Like to listen to your voice.
I can't forget you.
I hope you will talk to me.

Why?

I love you.
Let me tell you about myself.

I was as silent as the Great Wall of China.

Frank tried to tell me
when he was born,
how many brothers and sisters he had,
how his father and mother were,
what they did for a living,
what sort of an education he had received.
Every night for a month,
he called from Chicago.

Then letters came.
Some shared his poems to me;
others told me about his education
to become an airline pilot.
All expressed his love for me.

I think he is a mental case,
I confided to Dutsen.

Well, let's see what Professor Yin has to say,
Dutsen unsympathetically replied.

Professor Yin from Shanghai Medical College?
I beamed, thoroughly pleased and surprised.

Dutsen quietly nodded.

What is he doing here?

He's in New York for a conference.
I invited him here for dinner tonight.

At dinner we reminisced
about Shanghai Medical College.

I remember the Japanese soldiers
kicking their nurses,
shuddered Dutsen.

Mrs. Cara was so good to me,
I recalled.
Let me work
in the Chinese concentration camp.
She could have used
her supervisory power,
could have said,

"As you are well aware, Miss Chu,
I am short-staffed.
We need good nurses
at Shanghai Medical College.
You need to learn to get tough."
Instead, she chose to let me follow
my good judgment.

Dr. Yin, I have some problems,
Dutsen changed the topic.
I cannot make Cho-Shin understand
that a certain man truly likes her.
He continues to call her,
writes her letters.
She doesn't respond.

Could I read his letters?
Dr. Yin gently asked me.

Oh, she wants you to read them,
interjected Dutsen.
I do, too.
I don't know
why she thinks he is a mental case.

I don't care what you do,
I resisted.
I have no feeling.

A thorough person,
Dr. Yin poured
over each letter,
weighing carefully one
with the other.

After careful consideration,
he concluded,
I can understand
how you think, Mabel,
considering the way you grew up
and how you were educated.

According to these letters, however,
I think Frank is sincere,
not a mental case.

His letters are all focused.
Writing is good.
He aims to share his feeling for you,
and he does.
Why didn't you answer?

I don't know
where I'm going to be.
I don't want
 to become too entwined.
I don't want
to begin a relationship
that might have to end.

You worry too much,
consoled Dr. Yin.
You should know Frank
a little better.
My advice to you is
to answer him.
He's so far away.
He can't kill you.

We laughed.

He spends money to give you a good time,
cajoled Dr. Yin.
You don't appreciate?

True,
I had forgotten genuine courtesy.

Dear Frank,
I wrote,
I feel guilty.
What did I do to deserve
this kind of friendship?
I might have to leave this country
some time soon.
If I can stay here,
I would like to find a job.
I must see Father Reese first.
Sincerely,
Mabel

The telephone rang one evening.

Hello,
I answered.

If you and I become friends,
Frank began,
at least let us talk a little.
Tell me your problems.
I may be able to help.

I realize
I shouldn't stay
in my friend's house too long,
I confided.
Either I go to Taiwan
or to San Francisco
to see Father Reese.
The reason I hesitate
to go to San Francisco
is because I don't think working
for just room and board is worthwhile.
I don't want to be just a housekeeper.
I came to this country
to learn anesthesia.
I have a strong feeling
anesthesia is my life's work.
Yet, if I go to San Francisco,
my train travels via Chicago.

Oh, you may come to Chicago?
Frank anticipated.
If you can come to Chicago for a short time,
I'll be able to tell you more about who I am,
what I am,
how I love you.
I think it is meant to be.

Will you rent a room for me
at the YWCA?
For two days?

It was March 1949.
I planned to stay in Chicago
only a couple of days.

30

Here's where you are staying,
hosted Frank.
Five blocks to my restaurant this way,
five blocks to Lincoln Park that way.
Tomorrow we'll go to the art museum,
see the Asian art.
By the way,
did you think about
us getting married?

How could I?
I cannot stay in this country,
unless I work.

It is always easy to find a job.
Do you have a job in San Francisco?

I came to this country
to learn anesthesia,
I repeated.
If I cannot learn anesthesia,
then I should go to Taiwan.
Perhaps I could return sometime.

If we become engaged,
it would be different,
offered Frank.

I don't know you very well.
My father would not like me
to become divorced.
Seems like there are
too many divorces in America.

Don't talk that way,
discouraged Frank.
You don't know me,
but I know me.

We should get to know each other soon.
I reserved a room here at the Y
for five days.

Why didn't you tell me
you wanted me to stay longer?

I want you to know me better.
I'll see you tomorrow.

I could hardly say *no.*

When Frank returned,
he brought part of his library.
Here are my five books
about aeronautical engineering
that I translated into Chinese.

Completely bewildered,
I accepted his treasures,
I thought you studied to become a pilot.

I did.
But I have mild color-blindness.
I translated these, hoping to return
to the University of Shanghai.
Since we met, maybe we'll return
to China together.

Since the Japanese War,
the Chinese economy is not good.
I don't think you could adjust.

My mother didn't want to come
to the United States,
Frank continued, undeterred.

If we go to Shanghai,
maybe she could stay with us.

He checked his watch,
I must return to my restaurant,
replace an ill waitress.
You think about it.

And so he left me
to read all those books.

I like you,
I know
I'll love you forever,
Frank continued his proposal
for the second day.
I hope you will have
a little feeling for me.
Is that enough?

Which book should I read first?

Do you think
you could have
a little feeling for me?

I'll try.

Oh, thank you.
I'll call Mrs. Graham.

Who is Mrs. Graham?

Oh, she's my good friend,
George Graham's mother.
George and I trained to be pilots.

An engagement party was arranged
by George and Mrs. Graham.
I wrote to my brother:
I met a man here
 who is Cantonese.
I don't know
 if we can get along or not.
My English is not good.
This gentleman, Frank, promised
he would help me with English,
and I promised
I would help him
to speak Mandarin.
Don't you think
this is a good exchange?

Nine days later,
I received my brother's letter.

Frank,
here is a clipping
of our engagement
in the Shanghai newspaper.

My brother writes:
"I wish I could meet Frank.
You are independent now.
You do what you think is right.
I wish I could see both of you."

Sounds like him,
I reflected, still amazed.
When I wished to follow
the Christian faith, he said,
"You are going to be independent.
You do what you think is right.
Just don't try to change my way.
I must follow in my father's footsteps."

This letter was almost
my brother's last to me.
After the war began,
we had no way to connect.
In 1986, when I returned
to China for the first time,
I learned that my brother
had been abused,
sent to Siberia
for hard labor.
So much of what we learn
is after the fact.

At that time,
I didn't know Frank was ill.
After our engagement party,
Frank's unhealed stomach ulcer
began to bleed.
After we married,
April 18, 1949,
Frank had a heart attack due
to an overdosed blood transfusion.*

*According to Dr. David Williams, Chinese physicians effectively used the roots of
rhubarb to treat bleeding ulcers.

I began to work in the restaurant
when Frank could not.

One evening, when I returned home,
Frank pleasantly surprised me,
What?
Painting a whole bed sheet?

Many scenes, one moment!
enjoyed Frank.
Mountains, a stream, a pagoda,
two men talking in a gazebo,
some trees.

Who taught you to paint like that?

My uncle.
He was a famous painter.
He passed on the art to me
when I turned fourteen. *

That was four years
before you came to this country.

Yes, I came here in 1929
when I was eighteen.
My father wanted me
to have permanent residence
as an immigrant.

During the times Frank's ulcer bled,
he stayed home at length to paint.*

---

*Frank practiced one of the classical Chinese medical arts, the landscape painting of harmony and balance emergent from Chinese calligraphy. According to the contemporary Chinese calligrapher and brush painter, Professor Wang, Gongyi, continued practice of these arts for a long time can improve physical health and spiritual life. This is because these arts help us to center our *qi* or vital energy, calm our minds, focus on our innermost being, and understand nature through experience and observation. Each of the five fingers used (or unused) to hold and turn the brush corresponds to one of five elements and one of five vital organs. According to a seventeenth generation qigong master, Zhongxian Wu, a contemporary Chinese calligrapher recovered from a stroke by continuing his practice. The Jungian analyst and hypnotherapist, Ernest Rossi, accounts for this phenomenon with new neuroscience hypotheses offered in his recent book, ***The Psychobiology of Gene Expression***.

Much later, Frank gave me a painting
on white satin.
Today I painted
something for both of us.
Since I'm feeling better now,
hopefully we can be together more.
You've been so good to me.

Frank narrated,
Your name is Bamboo.
I didn't know
if I could draw bamboo or not.
Yet I wanted to draw our story.
So, here is bamboo branch.
On branch are two birds.
One has closed eyes, resting.
That's me.
The other is singing,
making my life enjoyable.
That's you.
Seems like these two
get along fine.

We laughed.

Read the characters to me,
I demanded like a youngster.

Honorable people
are not afraid of poverty.

31

Frank's ulcer continued to bleed
every three to five months.
I wrote to my friend,
Dr. Janet Wong,
Dear Janet,
Frank's doctor wants him to rest
in Arizona where the climate is dry
and the life style quieter than Chicago.
Could we come to see you before?
We don't know how long we'll be in Arizona.
Love,
Mabel

Janet's response arrived soon,
Dear Mabel,
We welcome you.
You may stay as long as you like.
Love,
Janet

Ok, ok,
accepted Frank,
we go to Tennessee
to see Dr. Janet Wong
and her husband.
But first we go
to the Social Security Office.

Why?
What is Social Security?

You need it
to work in this country.
My first cousin has a hardware store
in Arizona.
Maybe
you can work there.

I hope
I don't have to work
in a hardware store,
I prayed.

Before long,
Frank sold his restaurant business,
and we traveled by train
to Tennessee
in September 1949.

32

You mean they live
right in the State Hospital
with their mental patients?
Frank asked in disbelief
as we rang the doorbell
of Dr. Janet Wong's
and Dr. Chen's home.

Yes,
I remained calm
and formal.

And this is where
we are going to stay, too?
worried Frank.

Yes,
I firmly replied.

I don't think
I'd like to live with—

Welcome! Janet hugged me.
Mabel, it's been so long.

Frank,
this is Dr. Janet Wong
and her husband, Dr. Chen,
I introduced.

Mabel tells me you three met
in Rochester,
Frank gracefully responded.

Yes, Janet glowed.
We met at a neighborhood grocery store.

I had left my purse there
the day before.
The grocer found it,
and I was just saying thank you
when Janet and her husband walked in.

There were few Chinese in Rochester
at that time,
recalled Janet.

There are few Chinese in Tennessee
at this time,
compared Dr. Chen.

We lived two blocks apart,
I recollected.

Well, come in,
come in, invited Janet.
Please make yourselves at home.

How did you decide to live in Tennessee?
Frank wondered.

Mayo did not permit couples
 to work together,
replied Dr. Chen.
Janet worked in GYN
at Northwestern University Hospital in Chicago,
while I practiced psychology at Mayo.

I returned to Rochester twice a month.
That's twenty-four hundred miles!
Janet marveled.

When we learned
we could practice together
here in Tennessee,
we were grateful,
smiled Dr. Chen.

We began our practice here
about the same time Mabel left
Rochester for New York,
remembered Janet.

We corresponded
between Tennessee and New York,
I explained.
I told them about our engagement, Frank.

About my being—
Frank hesitated.

We knew about your marriage
and your living in Chicago,
continued Janet.
We didn't know,
until recently,
about your illness, Frank.

Oh, I bounce back ok.
Go to the hospital
four or five days;
then I'm right back to work,
minimized Frank.

Janet and I exchanged looks.

He is not supposed
to work at all now,
I tried not to exaggerate.

Well, you two please stay here
as long as you like,
Janet warmly encouraged.
We're looking forward
to your long visit.

Shall we share dinner now?
hosted Dr. Chen.

When we are together,
we are always eating,
aren't we?
noticed Janet.

With Janet and her husband,
Frank and I felt at home.
They gave us much time alone,
let us make our own breakfasts.

Not long after our arrival,
Janet's friend, Dr. Baker,
wished to speak with me,
Mrs. Tow, are you going to settle
in Arizona?

Yes, we plan to.

I was thinking
how good it would be
for you to live here
where you have friends close by.
You would be good for Dr. Wong
and her husband, too.

I'd like you to be a surgical nurse here.
We have some surgeries,
not much,
but right now, we select
nurses from general duty.
As you know, we provide
room and board.
How much salary would you like to have?

I think
I have to talk
to my husband.

I walked from the telephone
to the breakfast table,
Frank,
Janet's friend, Dr. Baker,
would like us to live here.
He asked me to be a surgical nurse.
What do you think?

You have a sick husband.
I don't think I'd like
for you to work with mental patients.
I don't think I'd like
to live here.

Immersed in warm hospitality
and friendship,
Frank and I continued to stay
over a month in Tennessee.
Dr. Baker telephoned again,
Mrs. Tow, I have good news to tell you.
Maybe you would like to work in surgery
at the new Jackson hospital.
This new hospital just opened last October.
They don't have enough surgical nurses.
One is on leave-of-absence.
When I asked if they would need a surgical nurse,
they said, "Oh, for sure."
So I made an appointment
for you to meet them.

Dr. Baker found a job for me in Jackson!
My enthusiasm spread.

Wonderful! Janet jumped up.

I hope you can get this job,
Frank readily accepted.
We'll go to Jackson right away.

Thank you, Dr. Baker,
I returned to the telephone.

The new hospital is only fifteen minutes by bus.
Your interview is with Carrie McCasko.

33

As Frank and I exited the bus,
he noticed,
The neat looking policemen,
clean streets, calm atmosphere,
all impress me.
Jackson must be
a well-organized city.

He sat down on the park bench
outside the hospital
and opened the local newspaper,
I'll wait for you here.

Carrie McCasko met me with graciousness,
and our interview went so well that,
when I returned, I decided to be a little naughty to Frank,
I'm back already.
Let's catch the next bus home.

Not waiting for his answer,
I continued walking to the bus stop.
Frank walked close behind,
Did you get the job?
Did you?
Mabel, did you get the job?
. . . Well, did you?

How American Frank had become.
I tried to temper his soaring spirit,
return it to its Chinese levity,
able to accept good and bad fortune alike.

Did you get the job, or didn't you?

I got the job.
Carrie McCasko employed me right away.
But!

But?

I have to work
as a general duty nurse
for the first four months.
What do you think?

I found a house for rent

"I found a house for rent."
That was Frank's way
of masking and revealing his delight.
He, too, was glad
I didn't have to work
in a hardware store.

We explored the house with levity.
I've never seen a house like this one,
all open underneath the porch
to let cats and dogs and who knows
what else run through,
I inspected.
The neighborhood is pretty rundown.

Designated for Negroes
according to the realtor,
informed Frank.
We would be the first Chinese tenants.

Inside is clean, I found,
simple, but not new or inviting.
Walls need fresh paint,
new wallpaper.
I don't know.
For a hundred dollars a month—
I hesitated.

We'll take it,
Frank decided.

Between hospital admissions
every three to five months,
Frank continued to paint.
He also managed an import shop
in our home.
His cousin in Hong Kong supplied
intricately carved ivory and china statues.

I had worked with Jackson Hospital staff
for a year, when the ANA
(American Nurses' Association) visited,
Hello, Mabel.
I'm Nina Wootton,
Secretary Consul of the ANA.
I'm pleased to meet you.
Carrie has told me
what a good surgical nurse you are.

She even cleans all the instruments,
Carrie praised.

I'm here to evaluate nursing care,
Nina explained.
Thank you, Mabel,
for bringing Carrie your nursing diploma.

We watched her read through the diploma.

Oh, it's signed
by Elizabeth Riley,
recognized Nina.
Elizabeth and I are good friends.
Mabel's nursing education must have been
excellent, since Elizabeth Riley supervised it.
Can we call her?

Yes, assured Carrie.
I'll dial.

I just need to learn more
about the credentialing process
at your school, Mabel,
Nina interpreted.

Hello.
Mrs. Riley?
This is Carrie McCasko, calling
from Jackson Hospital in Tennessee.
A friend of yours, Nina Wootton, is here
and would like to speak with you.
She handed the receiver to Nina.
Now don't you worry, Mabel, honey.
As I told you,
this is a routine visit from the ANA,
pure and simple.

Mabel is not only an R.N.,
Nina affirmed,
she is a national honor R.N.

Now, why didn't you tell me that, Mabel?
Carrie scolded good-naturedly.

Mabel, continued Nina,
based on your credentialing in China,
we can award you an American R.N.

I was so surprised.
Continue to wonder how it is
I have today,
why God has been so good to me.

I must remember my angels,
Elizabeth Riley, Janet Wong, Dr. Baker, and Carrie McCasko.

Janet, a naturally compassionate person,
never took credit for introducing me to Dr. Baker.
Dr. Baker, so happy to encourage Chinese friends to be neighbors,
always expressed good will.
His good will to his staff
impressed me beyond words.
And Carrie, who always praised my work,
gave me a job,
which would benefit Frank in his illness.
Carrie was instrumental
in my American credentialing
and my eventual self-reliance.
God must have chosen these people
to be in my daily life.

Otherwise, I could not have kept my path,
followed in my father's footsteps.

One evening,
when I returned home from work,
Frank looked up from his painting,
There's an article in this evening's newspaper about you.

About me?
Why?
All I could remember
was the **Rochester Post Bulletin** article
and Mr. Hansen, the immigration officer.

Just read it,
Frank encouraged.
I left the paper on the kitchen table.
It's opened to the right page.

New surgical nurse
from China joins
Jackson Hospital staff,
I read aloud.
Surgeons report
that she is very capable.
They are happy
to have her practice with them.
Before moving to Jackson,
Mrs. Mabel Chu Tow worked at Mayo.

Well, that's nice.
Didn't expect any publicity.

A Mrs. Jeannie Murdock telephoned,
Frank added.

Mrs. Jeannie Murdock?
I questioned.

Yes.
Sounds elderly.
Said she'd call back for you.

Wonder what kind of an old lady
would want to bother me?

The telephone rang.
Hello.
Yes, this is Mrs. Tow.
. . . Mrs. Jeannie Murdock?
Do we know each other from somewhere?
. . . You want to meet me?
. . . Mrs. Mary Lynch will call for me tomorrow?
Bring me to your house?
Is it ok?

I couldn't say *no.*

The following afternoon,
when I answered the doorbell,
Mary offered me her hand,
Hello, I'm Mrs. Mary Lynch.

Pleased to meet you,
I accepted her hand.
We stood for a time
in uncomfortable silence.

Finally, Mary spoke,
May I sit with you a moment?
Let me tell you why Mrs. Murdock wants to see you.

Oh, I'm so sorry.
Didn't invite you in.
Please—

Mrs. Murdock loves Chinese people,
Mary confided as we moved inside.
Her sister trained to be a missionary to China.
You are Chinese, aren't you?

Yes.

Did you know any Chinese here before coming to this country?

No.
I came here to take
special training at Mayo.

May I take you to meet Mrs. Murdock now?

Is it necessary?

Is it necessary?
Mary repeated my question.
She had to think how to answer me.

*Oh, you don't **know** Mrs. Murdock,*
she finally realized.

Never heard of her,
I honestly responded.

Everybody in Jackson admires Mrs. Murdock,
***wants** to get to know her.*

Again, I couldn't say *no.*

It was November 1951,
and I enjoyed autumn colors
as we drove to Mrs. Murdock's home,
a large mansion with a fish pond
in downtown Jackson.

Unpretentious, Mrs. Murdock,
a woman close to eighty,
tall and slim,
met us at the door,
You must be Mabel Chu Tow.
Welcome, dear.
Come in and share some tea with me.
How's Frank's trouble?

He has coped with an ulcer
since we've been married.

Dr. Leland Johnston,
my physician,
told me Frank is very ill.
What do you think?

He can't continue this way.
We have to consider surgery,
possibly a resection.

Well, the doctors here are good.
Our Dr. Johnston is head cardiologist at Jackson Clinic.
His practice is well-respected, not only by his patients,
but by the sixteen doctors who own the clinic.
How did you decide to stay in Jackson?

I shared my story
as best I could,
beginning with my aim to study
anesthesia at Mayo
and meeting my good friend,
Dr. Janet Wong in Rochester.

Oh, I've been a Mayo patient, too.
Mrs. Murdock shared.
A long time ago, I stayed in Mayo's home.
Their horse and carriage took me to and from the clinic.
I think you and I have a deep, inner connection.
My whole family thinks Chinese people are wonderful.
My sister studied to be a missionary to China.
I want to do what I can for you, while you are here.
Can we be friends?

Later, I learned how
Mrs. Murdock had taken
many young boys under her wing,
sent them to college to receive a good education.
She had helped one in particular
to open a flower shop in Jackson.
Before I left her home
that afternoon of our first meeting,
she tucked forty dollars into my hand,
Find something for Frank.
I hope we can see each other often.

34

Frank avoided surgery
as long as possible.
Dr. Johnston met me
outside his hospital room,
Because of Frank's cardiac condition,
a stomach resection could be a high risk operation.
Do you think Frank would want to go to Mayo?

Let's ask him.

Frank, how are you today?
Dr. Johnston asked.

I have Mabel
to take care of me now.
We're happy.
I think I'll be ok.

Well, we've avoided that stomach resection as long as possible.
Mabel and I wonder whether you'd like to go to Mayo for your surgery.

I think I'll be ok,
Frank repeated.
Mabel and I will talk.

I recently met
another of your patients,
Dr. Johnston,
I confided.

Wouldn't be Jeannie Murdock, would it?

How did you know?

Mrs. Murdock visited me
with that newspaper article about you in hand,
"Is it true? Is it true?"
"Totally."
"How can she do what she does?"
"Well, her English isn't good,
but she can perform nursing duties
better than anyone here."
That's true, Mabel. That's true.
Yes, Jeannie is a real character.
She has two physicians,
me and a friend's doctor.
I pretend not to know.
Just say, "Oh, you're taking different medications now."

We laughed.

She called me,
I shared.

"I want to meet you."
Didn't know what to say.
Just couldn't say no.

With the same patience
he gave to Jeannie Murdock,
Dr. Johnston met Frank
and Frank's fear of surgery.
Eventually, Frank agreed to schedule
a resection at Jackson Hospital.

One morning, an LPN,
obviously new to her job,
brought into Frank's room
an armload of bath towels.

You're not here again
to give me a bath,
are you?
Frank protested.

Well, yes. You must. Baths are part of your daily care,
defended the LPN.

But I don't want you
to give me a bath,
roared Frank
in his crabbiest disposition,
frightening away the LPN.

Carrie McCasko introduced you
to three good nurses,
an R N and two LPNs,
I reprimanded.
"Let him choose
who he would like,"
she offered.
You don't appreciate?

I don't know them,
Frank defended.

*You don't have to **know** them!*
You are a patient,
I reminded.

I still don't know
if Frank couldn't choose,
or wouldn't.
He acted like a Chinese girl
introduced to three strange suitors.

Only Dorothy Evans,
another of my angels,
could cajole Frank out
of an ill humor.
Dorothy was supervisor
of the medical section
at Jackson Hospital
and our good friend.
Often invited to our house
for dinner,
Dorothy always praised
Frank's six-course meals.
Dorothy was the only nurse
who could give Frank a bath.

Good morning, Frank.
I thought I'd say hello before my shift begins.

Pretty early.
6 a.m.
Good morning, Dorothy.

I miss your wonderful six-course dinners, Frank.

Looks like you came
to give me a six-course bath.

That's right.
I'm the only one here, who gives six-course baths.

Every morning
until Frank's death,
Dorothy would visit,
give Frank a bath,
put fresh linens on the bed,
and dress him in a clean gown.
Couldn't forget my angel, Dorothy.

35

Shortly before surgery,
Frank suffered another heart attack.

Mabel,
are you there?

I held his head in my arms.

If I die in your arms,
I'll be happy.
But I'm not going to die.
I'm going to be with you.
Don't worry,
don't worry.
Mabel,
if I die—

Don't think about that now.

Frank raised his hand
to touch my face,
Mabel—
Then his head rolled to the side.

February 18, 1952
(two years, ten months
after we were married)
Frank died.

Mrs. Murdock was right there
to take me to the funeral home.
I was shocked.
Hadn't thought about burying him.

After Frank's death,
Dorothy came to visit me often,
How are you doing, Mabel?

Just sent eighty dollars
to Frank's mother in Hong Kong.
Four months ago,
we sent her three hundred.

I've saved five hundred
from Dr. Ting's twenty-two-hundred,
just enough to bury Frank.
Mrs. Murdock said
we could bury Frank
in her family ground.
I was shocked.
Turned out,
the whole cemetery belongs
to the Murdock family.

We laughed.

Now she wants to adopt me.
"Just call me Aunt Jenny."
I never dreamed anyone like her.
I can't let her adopt me.
I don't know
whether or not
I can stay in the U.S.
Besides, I don't want
to burden someone her age.

Oh, you wouldn't be a burden.
You come to my place after dinner tomorrow night, ok?

I don't know.
Tomorrow
I go to the immigration office in Memphis
to apply for a green card.

Oh, hadn't you better let me or Miss Hansen go with you?

No, I must do
something for myself.
Can't always be
dragging you away
from your work.

Dorothy had a husband
and four children to tend.
Yet she never left me
without inviting me
to her place for dinner.

Now, I have one huge album
of all of her grandchildren.

Dorothy and Miss Hansen found me
exiting the immigration office in Memphis.
We're so glad we found you,
they chimed in unison.
Both hugged me at once.

Shhhhh!
Everyone is looking,
I blushed.

We thought you might be lost,
Miss Hansen admitted
as I struggled out of their arms.

I have to be independent.
Learn to do things by myself.

Well, we know than, hon',
Miss Hansen continued.
We came to put our own minds at ease.

Look.
Even the immigration officer
is looking at us now.

Let's go to my place for dinner,
Dorothy ended the little scene.
I'll drive us all home.

Even at that time,
Mrs. Murdock was entertaining
ideas of moving to Rochester with me
and of buying a house for us to live in
so that I could continue to study anesthesia.
Within ten days,
Mayo responded
to my letter of July 1952,
Dear Mrs. Tow,
We have an opening in anesthesia in October.

Just like a dream.
A dream.

I see now the pattern
in which I lived.
If I hadn't met
my future husband in New York,
I would have gone from New York
to Washington, D.C.
to San Francisco
to Taiwan,
perhaps never to return,
perhaps never to learn anesthesia.
How could I forget Frank?
My angel, Frank Tow.

Dear Mrs. Tow,
Mrs. Murdock repeated the letter from Mayo.
We have an opening in anesthesia in October.
She gave me a hug,
Oh, I'm real glad for you, honey, real glad.
Mayo is a good place.
Here, sit down, have some good Chinese tea with me.
She poured two cups.

I've been thinking,
I reflected.

Yes, honey,
Mrs. Murdock reflected with me.

I have to be independent,
do things for myself.

Of course you do, of course.
I've rethought my plan.
We can't move to Rochester.
I thought earlier we could, but my sister—
You know how deaf and nearly mute she is.
She's still attached to home here in Jackson.
With her limitations, a move to Rochester would be too much.
Yet I want you to be the best you can be at Mayo.
So here's what I'm going to do.
I'm going to give you a thousand dollars to buy a car.

A car?

You can learn to drive and be on your own in Rochester.
How does that sound?

To think Mrs. Murdock placed
my welfare before her sister's
astonishes me.
Jeannie Murdock really wanted
what was right for me.
Jeannie, my angel, helped me
to continue in my father's footsteps.

36

During my first three months
back at St. Mary's,
I worked in general surgery.
My evenings were spent
studying anesthesia
under Dr. Roger W. Ridley's supervision.
A senior student,
Mr. Erickson and I
were sometimes teammates.

How do you like studying with Dr. Ridley?
Mr. Erickson asked me
after we had just given
a patient anesthesia.

He's very thorough.
Always asks each of us
three or four questions
every class.

Sounds just like him.
He always drilled us, too.

He's not as stern as Dr. Pender.

Yeah,
agreed Mr. Erickson,
most students are afraid of Dr. Pender.
He's a man of few words.
If you ask him a question though,
he's always patient and gives a thorough answer.
Otherwise, he doesn't converse with students.

Mabel,
interrupted Dr. Ridley,
will you go to Uro
to relieve staff for lunch?

Yes, Dr. Ridley.

I heard him to say *Neuro*
instead of *Uro.*
Minutes later,
I reported back,
Dr. Ridley,
Ruth Bozikowski told me
she didn't need any relief in Neuro.

I told you to go to Uro!

Mr. Erickson stifled a laugh
as I rushed off to Uro.
Uro didn't need relief either.

After three months,
I was scheduled
to work in orthopedics
under Dr. Pender.
Dr. Pender had heard the story
about Neuro-Uro confusion,
no doubt from Dr. Ridley.

Mrs. Tow,
I think it would be good for you to look for another job,
since your English is inadequate,
Dr. Ridley dismissed me.

Thank you,
I accepted.
I thought it was
my last day
in anesthesia.

Dr. Pender visited
when I was giving anesthesia
to my last patient,
Mr. Erickson,
how is Mrs. Tow doing?

*Ok. **This** is her fourth patient today.*

Dr. Pender then pondered my report,
Report looks good.
Mabel, you do all right.

I think I do ok,
but I'm going to say
good-bye to you.

Why?
Dr. Pender looked
mildly surprised.

Dr. Ridley told me to leave.

Why?
persisted Dr. Pender.

Dr. Ridley doesn't think
I'm able to learn anesthesia.

Why?
Dr. Pender gently asked.

My English.

What do you think, Mr. Erickson?

I think she's ok.
She's not been here even six months.

Ok,
concluded Dr. Pender.
When you finish your work today, Mrs. Tow,
come to my office.

What do I do next?
What do I do next?
My mind ticked like a metronome.

I'll clean house this evening, Mabel,
offered Mr. Erickson.
You go see Dr. Pender.

We better say
good-bye,
I responded.

The short hallway
to Dr. Pender's office
seemed like that subway
wherein long ago
I became lost.

Dr. Pender,
I'm here,
I announced.
I want to say
good-bye to you.

Why?

Dr. Ridley told me
early this morning
not to come back tomorrow.
Thought I should best
look for another job.

Will you go to Dr. Ridley?
Give him a message for me?
Dr. Pender was so patient.

I'll try.

Tell Dr. Ridley,
if Dr. Deveroe can be staff,
Mrs. Tow can be a trainee.

You want me to say this?

Yes, tell Dr. Ridley,
Dr. Pender told you
to tell him this.

Later, I learned
that Dr. Deveroe always spoke
with a thick, Belgian accent.
But at the time,
I was totally innocent.

You! Are you going?
barked Dr. Ridley.

Dr. Pender told me
to tell you
if Dr. Deveroe can be staff,
Mrs. Tow can be trainee.

Ok,
Dr. Ridley calmed down,
if John said so,
you stay.

Dr. Pender is
how I have today.

Like my other angels' strange kindness,
Dr. Pender's kindness allowed me
to continue in my father's way.

37

Dr. Ting called me in 1978,
I have just returned
from Siberia—
hard labor.
I'd like to rebuild
my hospital in Shanghai.
Could you return
to help?

I've just retired.
My blood pressure is high,
could have a stroke.
I retired out of concern
for my patients.
Should I have a stroke
and my patient die because of me,
I could not be happy with myself.
How can I justify returning
to Shanghai now?
Let me send you some money.

That would be fine,
Dr. Ting graciously accepted.

Can you also send me
a bottle of One-A-Day
Multiple Vitamins?

We laughed.

Dr. Ting died, rebuilding
his dream.

I cannot return
his generosity.

As keen as my suffering is,
my memory is as vivid
of Dr. Ting returning to Shanghai
from Rochester in 1947
to tell me about Sr. Mary Brigh
and St. Mary's postgraduate course.

Here's twenty-two hundred dollars.
I'm going to send you over there as your vacation
because of your hard work.

My brother won't be happy.
We've not seen each other since the war.

You'll be gone only two years.
We'll see about getting your visa
and someone to teach you English.

I couldn't say any more
about my brother.

Many people guided me in my life's way
to follow in my father's footsteps.
Why?
I don't know.
I tell people this story
many times.
I still don't know.
It is a mystery.

Leaves wave slowly on their branch,
Clouds flow around,
Fragrant wind touches my face.
        Oh, wind, could you touch my friends far away?
        *Give them my soft words? ***

*Tow's *soft* echoes verse 78 from the **Tao Te Ching** attributed to Lao Tzu. Stephen Mitchell translates: *Nothing in the world/ is as soft and yielding as water. / Yet for dissolving the hard and inflexible, / nothing can surpass it. / The soft overcomes the hard; / the gentle overcomes the rigid.*

PART TWO

Kindness in Words Creates Confidence

a commentary by Guangying Zhou

To live content with small means; to seek elegance rather than luxury, and refinement rather than fashion; to be worthy, not respectable, and wealthy, not, rich; to listen to stars and birds, babes and sages, with open heart; to study hard; to think quietly, act frankly, talk gently, await occasions, hurry never; in a word, to let the spiritual, unbidden and unconscious, grow up through the common—this is my symphony.
                                                        -William Henry Channing

Like others who will read ***Strange Kindness***, I wish I had known Mabel Chu Tow. Nevertheless, I feel immensely grateful to know her story in her own words. What a gracious example of compassion, humility and tenacity her life is. It is my sincerest hope for her story to be an inspiration to others, so that they may find their true calling so that they can be of service to humanity. As her life exemplifies, this is done through the simplest daily interactions.

At times our own light goes out and is rekindled by a spark from another person. Each of us has cause to think with deep gratitude of those who have lighted the flame within us.
                                                        –Albert Schweitzer

In this way, she reminds me of the many great teachers in my studies of Classical Chinese Medicine. It hasn't been simply the knowledge or pearls of wisdom that they have dispensed that have been so valuable. Much of this can be found in some book. Far greater has been their example. There is some transmission that occurs between great masters and anyone observing them, listening to them, attending not only to what they say, but to what they leave out. Attending the transmission has been an integral part of our training in the Classical Chinese Medicine tradition, and Dr. Chu Tow proves to be a great master, transmitting her teaching through her story. Her story touches our hearts and makes us better people, and in the process, better healers.

Because this story is conversational, we also receive a sense of Dr. Chu Tow's heart. Even with only the most basic understanding of the adversity she must have gone through in China, due to her rank and gender and the hardships known to many immigrants to this country, it is easy for us to imagine that she could have told a story that was a litany of injustice, cruelty, and oppression. Instead we hear of her angels, her gratitude, her destiny opening up before her however slowly. There is no regret that it all did not happen faster. There is instead a recounting of so much kindness bestowed, and we hear from others how Dr. Chu Tow was then able to bestow kindness to others, to the poor, to her husband, to children, and even to a praying mantis.

Kindness in words creates confidence.
Kindness in thinking creates profundity.
Kindness in giving creates love.
–Lao Tzu

Benevolence, Courage, Humility, and Keen Observation: Tow's Classical Chinese Medical Arts

a commentary by Charles Liu

Used correctly, the word qi means the foundation of courage, will and intention.

-Adeline Yen Mah
Watching the Tree

This essay reflects upon my friendship with Tow, her excellent memory of Classical Chinese Medicine, and her practice of qigong, which nurtures *qi, the life-force*, the foundation of benevolence, courage, humility, and keen observation, those intentions that inform her healing arts.

How I knew Mabel S. Chu Tow

Before my second career as a health educator, I was an electrical engineer, working during the early 1970's for the computer main-frame giant, IBM, in San Jose, California. When IBM relocated my job to Rochester, Minnesota in 1978, I accepted and moved my family, my wife and two young children, to this relatively small, mid-western town. Rochester, named after Saint Roch, the medieval saint of plague victims, was in 1978 primarily a Mayo medical and IBM community with few Chinese residents. Being Chinese, my wife and I welcomed acquaintance with Mabel Tow, recently retired from her career as a nurse-anesthetist. With Tow we shared one of the most common enjoyments of Chinese people in this country, planting flowers and growing vegetables. Tow and I occasionally shared our backyard harvests, exchanging seeds and produce. When better acquainted, we exchanged family stories.

Even today, the harsh events of Tow's life continue to trouble and to sadden me--the deaths of her parents before she was fifteen, the destabilizing environment of war-torn China, the turmoil of her post-graduate education and status in the United States, her disenfranchisement from China, her separation from her elder brother and remaining family, the illness of her husband, Frank Tow, and his death, ending their brief marriage, the uncertainty of her career in the United States. All these events contrast with her benevolent character, her devotion to truth and to the well being of others, compelling me to question conventional wisdom about fortune, predestination, and fate.

My second career as a health educator began in 1994, immediately after I accepted early retirement from IBM. I began to teach tai chi and qigong meditation, and I initiated my practice of Tuina Massage (Chinese Acupressure) at Integrative Therapies of Assisi Heights. Later, I learned that several years before my retirement, Tow had already moved to an apartment in Charter House, Mayo's retirement living complex. She sometimes invited us to join her for Sunday brunches. Charter House also became one of the sites where I offered my weekly tai chi classes. There, in a spatial exercise room full of about twenty enthusiastic participants, including Tow, I taught tai chi movements such as *White Crane Flaps Wings*, *Wave Hands like Clouds*, and *Monkey Retreats*, combined with simple qigong postures and abdominal breathing practices. To encourage participation every week, and to improve the circulations of students' qi and blood, I gave each attending student a brief Tuina Massage at the end of our class. Everyone seemed to enjoy and to appreciate both the tai chi and the ritual massage.

In 1997, Tow was transferred to an assisted living quarter of Charter House. I could sense her frustration and her disappointment after this undesired move, since it revealed to her that her mental and physical health were beginning to decline. Moreover, this forced move damaged her self-confidence. Her attendance at tai chi classes became irregular. Though I made special, after-class visits to her to encourage her and to offer her Tuina Massage, and though she made efforts to smile all the time, I could sense her sadness and then her depression.

Tow's excellent memory of Classical Chinese Medicine

During my visits, Tow told me many stories about how she learned Classical Chinese Medicine and qigong from her father, a physician in Hankow, China. Since Tow was more at ease and more psychologically connected with me when speaking Mandarin Chinese, we usually conversed in our native tongues. Her father had encouraged her to become a physician of western medicine because of not only her intelligence and her good memory, but her capacity to continue the legacy of classical Chinese physicians—the capacity to be a healer of life. Now, eighty years later, she still remembered common herbs and their medicinal usages.

She told me that eating more ginger roots could alleviate her shoulder pain or any inflammation in the body and that dandelion, the most hated weed on American lawns, could be used *to clear and resolve toxins*. Her terms exemplify the typical language and concepts of Classical Chinese Medicine used to describe symptoms related to fever, swelling, scorching redness, pain, suppuration, etc. She remembered that fennel, which we grew in our gardens many years ago, could warm the kidney and could dissipate cold, harmonize the stomach and rectify the qi. One stomach disharmony is indigestion due to over-eating, causing stomach qi to become sluggish. A simple household treatment is to boil a handful of fennel seeds in water to make a strong odorous soup.

Drinking fennel soup enables excessive gas in the digestive tract to be expelled. Tow knew these holistic, herbal approaches of Chinese medicine, because her father had taught her about herbs and their medicinal effects.

Occasionally we discussed acupuncture. Tow remembered the exact names of acupuncture points and understood their locations, their indications, and contraindications. By *contraindication* we mean that treating certain points may cause harmful, instead of healing effects on certain patients. For example, indications for stimulating *San-Yin-Jiao* (SP-6 of the Spleen Meridian) are irregular menstruation, dysmenorrheal, uterine bleeding, etc. However, stimulating this point on pregnant women may cause inadvertent miscarriages. Therefore, pregnancy is a contraindication for such stimulation.

Tow recognized, for example, *Feng-Chi* points (a.k.a. *Wind Pools*), the hollow areas below the occipital bone which, when stimulated, alleviate stiff neck and headache. The International Acupuncture Chart codes *Feng-Chi* as 'GB-20', meaning the twentieth point along the Gallbladder Meridian. Chinese physicians, besides offering acupressure therapy, would insert a fine needle into the GB-20 point to treat painful eyes or blurred vision and to relieve common cold symptoms, dizziness, and nasal obstructions.

During Tuina Massage, Tow remarked the Gao-Huang point (BL-43 or the Bladder Meridian) at the spinal border of the scapula. She said, *I hope my sickness qi will not be trapped into this point,* reflecting her understanding of the Chinese saying: *The sickness qi enters the Gao-Huang point.* This expression means that an illness has reached its final stage and that doctors may not be able to save the patient's life.

Tow also remembered the many indications for treating Bl-43 and the intended effects, which include strengthening lung qi, for weak lung qi may cause symptoms such as asthma, coughing, chest pain, and excessive sweating. She remembered well *Back-Shu* points, acupuncture points along two lines paralleling the sides of the spinal column. *Shu* means *transport*, and *Shu* points connect the qi energy of vital organs such as the heart, lungs, kidney, spleen, and stomach to the *Shu* points on the Bladder Meridian. Stimulation of these points on the back invigorates organic functions, improving overall health.

Such specialized knowledge of Classical Chinese Medicine formed one of the paradigms shaping Tow's perception and judgment when, as a nurse-anesthetist, she observed pathways of illness and health within her patients. As I reflect now upon my good fortune to have been the listener and appreciator of Tow's stories, I realize that her accurate, extensive, and vivid memory implies that the principles of Classical Chinese Medicine had made a deep impression upon her. These principles may have helped her not only to endure the extreme vicissitudes of her life, but also to integrate her life and her healing art with western practices.

The principles of Classical Chinese Medicine derive from the practice of qigong, the practice that nurtures the life force. Nurturing the life force, qigong engages humility and instills benevolence, courage, and a keen capacity to observe nature, all the intentions of mind needed to practice medicine. Examples of these intentions abound in *Strange Kindness* as Tow reflects upon the choices that intersected to support her to fulfill her father's dream for her life. Tow's humility opened her to understand how the Tao provides for everything and how much love and gentleness are given to all beings and to all existence. Embodiment of stillness gave her peace in adversity. From peace, emerged courage supported by a greater consciousness. Her keen observation and benevolent attunement to the energies and emotions of her patients were needed to apply pre-surgical suggestive technique, a way of guiding a patient's inner thoughts with psychological acumen. Such skills were needed to manage the stages of anesthesia and to instill hope, affecting a patient's vision of health and recovery from surgery. Therefore, I want to focus now upon how Tow's benevolence, courage, humility, and keen capacity to observe nature were nurtured by her early practice of qigong.

Classical qigong

Not an anesthesiologist, I cannot describe with accuracy intersections between Tow's practice of Classical Chinese Medicine and her practice of administering anesthesia. I can only reflect upon the practice of qigong, the practice of meditating with images, movements, and mudras to shape intentions of mind, which direct qi along healing pathways, and I can only suggest how such shaping could inform the anesthetist's practice, indirectly benefiting the patient.

Qigong is an ancient form of cultivating and strengthening our life-energy through deep breathing, moving postures, meditation and other mind-body-spirit approaches to directing the flow of qi. Qi, according to CCM, is the life-sustaining energy that permeates the universe and moves through and within human bodies. The Chinese characters themselves reveal how qigong is a healing art. The character for *qi* contains two radicals or roots. The lower radical depicts *rice*, the upper *steam*; together, these radicals refer to *warm steam rising from a heated pot of newly cooked rice, the energy of fire under water.* In contemporary usage, *qi* refers to the air we breathe or the vital energy flowing through the meridians of our bodies. The word *gong* refers to *cultivating.* Qigong cultivates the intentions of the mind that direct qi in harmonious, life-strengthening ways, ways that maintain the fire under water to produce the warm steam rising from a heated pot of newly cooked rice.

When the life force fills a person, the qi flows strongly and freely, optimally integrating yin and yang energies. He or she is able to lead a healthy, happy life style. Conversely, when there are impediments or insufficient life-energy within a person, yin and yang energies do not optimally integrate to produce one another. Then the person experiences lethargy, pain or sadness, and illness, all of which lead to life-threatening disease.

Qigong practitioners learn to observe flowing and unflowing qi within themselves and within others, and they learn to redirect qi, correcting imbalances.* Like tai chi, qigong is mindfulness or meditation through movement. Unlike tai chi, which requires continuous, fluid movement like water flowing in a river, qigong requires stillness in motion. Stillness in motion consists of standing or sitting postures, mudras, repetitive, gentle movement phrases, abdominal breathing, and self-massage. All engage and develop the inner-eye's capacity to observe energy flow.

Both tai chi and qigong benefit practitioners in similar ways. Physiological benefits include improved breathing, balance, coordination, leg muscle strength and joint flexibility. Psychological benefits include calmness, stress management, increased ability to focus, and relieved anxiety and depression.

A holistic, self-healing regimen, qigong aims to cleanse, fortify and smooth one's internal flow of qi and blood, while reconnecting that flow with the universal life force. This reconnection achieves what Chinese call *the union between heaven and earth.* This union engages one's openness or humility, one's transparency to receive the universal life force given to all. From this union, benevolence, courage, clarity of vision, and keen observation emerge.

Physicians of CCM regularly practiced qigong and recommended this practice to their patients. They realized how regular qigong practice can correct impeded or sluggish qi and blood circulation, both of which they considered to be the cause of most diseases, including tumors or cancers. Even today qigong is a form of preventive medicine, still practiced to prevent illness by promoting health.

Regular qigong practice by generations of qigong masters and physicians alerted them to recognize areas of darkness, areas of obstructed qi flow, and enabled them to use their spiritual and mental intentions to direct the flow of qi, that pure white mist or dew-like substance, along a patient's meridians to dissolve these dark stagnations. In fact, Tow's father's name, Dr. Chu, meaning *Fragrance of* Dew, recognizes his special quality of pure qi and his capacity to be a physician.

Spiritually and genetically inheriting Dr. Chu's special quality of qi and the capacity to be a physician, Tow learned first to cultivate her own vital energy. Her early learning of qigong also gave her a basis for understanding how qi optimally flows through meridians and a practice for using her benevolent intentions to restore, balance, and direct that flow within herself and others. Perhaps these skills were not lost upon St. Mary's patients, who, though lacking the education to name them, *always asked for Chu-Chu.* These skills could well have benefited Tow's surgical patients, supporting their life force before, during, and after surgery.

Implications

After 1978, when Tow retired, interest in Chinese medicine increased worldwide among the medical profession. Evidence was sought concerning the practice and effects of qigong. The Shanghai Higher Education Publishing Company videotaped Dr. Lin Hou-sheng, a qigong master at Shanghai Traditional Chinese Medicine Hospital, while he revived a comatose patient by using his qi-projecting fingers, called *sword fingers*, to send his external qi to the patient's Yin-Tang point, a.k.a., the third eye on the forehead. Lin is also known to have used his external qi to successfully engage the healing energies of many patients coping with spinal injuries, facial nerve palsies, and lumbar vertebrae fractures. A master's use of his or her external qi to treat patients is called in Chinese *Wai-Qi-Zhi-Liao*.

Not all qigong healings occur as dramatically as these renowned cases. Many ordinary qigong practitioners may use their intentions to emit their external energies, sending them to a patient's affected areas. Nonetheless, the patient's will to live is just as important as the healer's intention to heal. Volitions from our minds are subtle forms of healing energy, partly explaining, without the support of evidence collected by scientific method, how and why prayers have worked for over thousands of years. Further scrutiny of scientific study would only reinforce the efficacies of healing energies among ordinary people.

This essay has reflected upon my friendship with Tow, her memory of CCM, and how the medical art of qigong nurtures and cultivates the physician's intentions: benevolence, courage, humility, and a keen capacity to observe nature. Having recognized these intentions of mind within Tow and how they shaped her life and her career, I also recognize her among our long lineage of classical Chinese healers of life. I join her father, the first to witness her gifts, those natural and spiritual endowments indicative of life-purpose.

---

*Garret Yount's recent research suggests that when qigong masters transmit spiritual energy, their patients' body-cells entrain to the new wavelengths of light.

Reading *Strange Kindness* from Confucian and Taoist Perspectives

a commentary by Lily Tsang

Make of yourself a light.
-Buddha's last words

Every Chinese, it has been said, wears a Confucian thinking cap, a Taoist robe, and Buddhist sandals. This metaphor captures the three orientations toward being and reality that shape the Chinese mind, heart, and journey through life. This metaphor captures the three philosophies that shaped Tow's thought, her approach to life, and her awakening to the innate, noble heart of humankind. One of the first Chinese women to practice medicine in China and the United States, Tow nonetheless lived an exceptional life, one amazing to her witnesses. Though her story's significance will differ among readers, depending upon their viewpoints, that significance may be enhanced by an understanding of the guiding principles Chinese hold in common, the principles that guided Tow as she grew up to choose her own nature. A reader whose first language is Classical Mandarin, as was Tow's, and whose education focused upon Classical Chinese Literature, the major foundation of Classical Chinese Medicine, I will share those commonly held principles that shaped Tow's life in my reading of *Strange Kindness* from Confucian and Taoist perspectives.

Since Confucius and Lao Tzu taught their observations from nature, observations applied to cultivate the classical Chinese garden, and since Tow learned many of her early lessons in her father, Dr. Chu's classical garden, I invite the reader to enter *Strange Kindness* with me through the typical round, moon-shaped garden door. This door symbolizes reunion, completeness, and awakened spirit. A garden, at any time, is a small universe. There, we may observe natural law at work. There, we may also observe the delicate balance between nature and man-made elements, all mirroring the ancient Taoist virtue of human life lived in harmony with nature. By describing how a classical garden embodies and reflects the teachings of Confucius and Lao Tzu, I shall share how Tow's early learning was experiential and how the visual and metaphorical context of her education influenced her choices in later life.

The Confucian Thinking Cap

Upon entering a classical garden, we may notice the intersection of rectangular shapes: the rectangular classical Chinese house surrounded by separate, rectangular courtyards, all enclosed by a rectangular wall. The architecture regulates our path through the garden as well as to and from the house. Architectural regulation of human movement embodies Confucius's desire to regulate human interaction in relationships for the purpose of nurturing family, social, and political harmony.

Harmony in human relationships can be nurtured when individuals develop the virtues of loyalty, filial piety, fraternal love, and righteousness. These virtues shape five ideal relationships: relationships between emperor and officials, between father and son, between siblings, between husband and wife, and between friends. These virtues can be maintained when children give genuine respect to their elders and when elders give genuine care to their young. Each person, accordingly, contributes to universal harmony within his or her respective social position.

Confucius also observed how harmony flows best within relationships when people follow the middle way, avoiding excesses and deficiencies, both in their behavior and in their practice of *Li*, a series of mutually enacted, interpersonal rituals, such as the ritual of students and teachers bowing to one another.

Of all regulating principles, Confucius found benevolence or *Ren* to create the most harmony. Benevolence thereafter became viewed as the primary genial spirit and creative motive for practicing Chinese Medicine. Physicians, known as healers of life, were selected on the basis of both their intellectual capacity for medical expertise and their extraordinary benevolence, their capacity to realize the moral good and to express unselfish, natural love for people and all living creatures. *Ren Xing Ren Shu,* praise patients to honor the physician whose practice expresses the benevolence of *Zhong*, meaning *faithfulness*, and *Su*, meaning *forgiveness*.

Benevolence, then, was to permeate the classical Chinese garden just as it was to permeate the patient-physician relationship. Dr. Chu exuded benevolence, dedicating his practice to the poor who could not afford medical care. Benevolence was the primary virtue through which Dr. Chu inducted Tow into her future career. Benevolence was the primary virtue Dr. Chu cultivated within her.

Tow's exceptional memory, recognized by Dr. Chu's hired tutor, combined with her father's dream for her, a dream based upon her exceptionally benevolent nature, admitted her to a private education usually forbidden to the poor and to females of her generation. If, in rare cases, girls received any education, theirs was limited to study from the *Nu-Er-Jing*, a book dictating the ideal female role for their time. In the privileged environment of a private study and classical garden, Tow studied from age four to fifteen the fundamentals of Classical Chinese Medicine. The curriculum would have included calligraphy, qigong, Confucian books, the *Tao Te Ching*, the *I Ching*, *Hongfan*, *Huang Nei Jing*, and other medical books.

Among these books, *The Book of Three-Word Chants* was primary, rich in content stressing the importance of learning. With its outline and foundation rooted in Confucian teachings, the chants introduce beliefs of the great philosophers, knowledge of daily life, the elements in nature and the universe, the history of Chinese dynasties, and the practices of art. Tow recalls in *Strange Kindness* how her early education provided a strong foundation, enhancing her later academic expertise and professional medical career.

Strange Kindness reflects Tow's extraordinary benevolence. When Dr. Ting traveled abroad in 1947 to visit American hospitals, Tow secured the unity of their medical team by dispelling inharmonious ideas brewing in their ranks. Among their staff of twenty-one, nineteen strikers complained about two-dish meals and suffering, accusing Dr. Ting of receiving better treatment in the U.S. Tow reminded them with reasonable words: *Because of war, everyone has difficulty. Let's remember our benefits and Dr. Ting's care.* She showed the medical team their selfishness in unfounded accusations and led Dr. Ting's mission to bring the best possible medical care to the poor patients of war-ravaged China. In many other ways, Tow lived and was a witness to the discipline that Confucius emphasized most in human interactions: the discipline of keeping harmony among people.

Tow independently chose to follow in her father's footsteps and to combine eastern with western medical practices after opportunities and influences unfolded in her early life. Certain conditions, including a medical-family background, a tutor who recognized her giftedness, Dr. Chu's desire for her to step into his practice, an early education in Classical Chinese Medicine, and an elder brother who carried out his father's will, all arose in Tow's young life to guide her on a path divergent from others who were raised differently. All could have happened otherwise. Nevertheless, Dr. Chu, observant of his youngest daughter's healing gift, made certain choices in accord with her nature. Furthermore, Tow, in her independence, learned to prefer to act in harmony with her own nature. These choices reveal father's and daughter's Confucian thinking cap.

The Taoist Robe

Classical garden niches encourage meditation. Meditation nourishes the heart. The heart is the truth-seeking organ, according to the Taoist five-element practice of Chinese Medicine.

Taoists taught that to seek truth is to seek heaven and earth in all beings. Heaven and earth meeting in all beings may be found and contemplated in the classical Chinese garden's arrangement of yin and yang elements. Hard rock, a yang element, arranged in rock pilings symbolizes earth's structure. Taoists considered the heavenly rock on earth to be the home of the immortals. Soft water, a yin element, collected to form a lake, supports the lotus bloom, the yang fire of life, and balances with hard rock. Such interlinking of yin and yang elements mirrors the Taoist principle of harmony. To keep yin and yang, earth and heaven, in harmony is the major aim of Classical Chinese Medicine.

Taoist spirituality and practice are predominantly rooted in the teachings of the Yellow Emperor and Lao Tzu, a sixth and seventh century philosopher who observed the natural course of the universe and who practiced maintaining a tranquil mind. According to legend, Lao Tzu, in old age, left his post to travel to India. At the gateway of Hanguguan, he wrote down his wisdom on a scroll, which he gave to the gatekeeper. This scroll, gifted about 2,050 years ago, became known as the **Tao Te Ching**.

According to the **Tao Te Ching**, *Tao*, meaning *the way*, is the formless and nameless unifying virtue behind complex and contradictory happenings, the virtue that gives way to everything. Describing the Tao's series of natural births, Lao Tzu wrote in *chapter 42*: "The Tao gives birth to the One. / The One gives birth to the Two. / The Two gives birth to the Three. / The Three gives birth to every living thing." Every living thing holds yin and carries yang.

The book of **Zhouyi** linked relationships between yin and yang to the universe. Further study of yin and yang resulted in more books, such as the **Nei Jing**, which systematically analyzes the growing and fading of yin and yang in the human body.

Taoist understanding regarded yin and yang as opposing life-principles, which, though governed by the Tao, generate, then defeat each other. Accordingly, yin and yang may sustain one another by their resistance and tension. Tension or opposite conditions coexist within any circumstance. For example, within one tree root, growing and fading, growing and ceasing, ascending, descending, and transforming occur simultaneously. Within the human body, yin (cold) may transform into yang (heat) as when, in reaction to extremely cold weather, a person develops a heavy cold or flu with increasing fever. With their understanding of yin and yang, the ancient Chinese interpreted aspects of astronomy, meteorology, military, and medical science.

Taoists further described how combinations of heavenly odd numbers and earthly even numbers produce the five primary elements of fire, earth, metal, wood, and water. Because yin and yang coexist, the one always within the other condition, each gives birth to the other. Similarly, each element gives birth to another: metal gives birth to water, water to wood, wood to fire, fire to earth, and earth to metal. This cycle of birth produces, sustains, and destroys the elements, effectively balancing them, keeping the universe in existence.

The universe exists in miniature within each human body, according to Chinese medical science. Each miniature universe, each body, contains heaven and earth, and it is each person's responsibility to keep his/her yin and yang in balance. Whereas the materials of living organisms are considered the feminine, yin aspect of nature, the active functions of living beings are considered the masculine, yang aspect. The five yin organs of the body distribute active functions between them.

The heart or mind, referred to as the commander, controls consciousness and intelligence. Comparable to fire among the five primary elements, heart mind is vigorous in the season of summer. Lungs and respiratory system, responsible for cybernetic balance, regulate various bodily functions by oxygenating the blood. Comparable to metal, lungs are vigorous in the season of autumn. The liver regulates emotional response to the environment, actions of other organs, and the storage and balance of blood. Comparable to wood, the liver is vigorous in spring. The spleen, by distributing nutrition throughout the body, controls metabolism, bringing the body energy and strength. Comparable to earth, the spleen is vigorous in all four seasons. Kidneys store nutrition and energy. Comparable to water, kidneys are vigorous in winter. These five primary elements, five bodily organs, and four seasons of change in nature are all closely intertwined as described by Taoists.

Taoists also found the body affected by six, external disease-causing factors: wind, cold, heat, moisture, dryness, and internal heat. Excessive changes in weather may unbalance these factors and harm the body. In addition, Taoists discovered the body affected by seven, viscera-induced emotions: joy, anger, worry, pensiveness, grief, fear, and anxiousness. They observed how these seven emotions interact with the six external disease-causing factors to form the basis of disease. A Chinese physician can diagnose a patient's yin and yang deficiencies or excesses, determine the emotional and external disease-causing imbalances, and catalyze balance.

Balancing yin and yang, nourishing each, and keeping the viscera in rhythm with the life-force are so intrinsic to nature and to Chinese medical practice that Tow could not refrain from practicing Taoist medical art, regardless of harsh circumstances or Western medical contexts. Knowing that *nothing in the world is softer than water,* that *anything conquering hardness cannot be better than water,* Tow nourished the yin in her body. Such softness, she knew, could weather harsh circumstances, such as departure from St. Mary's Hospital, expulsion from China, and her husband, Frank Tow's illness and death. Such water-like softness could conquer toughness. Through water-like softness and through humility's openness, Tow overcame all difficulties challenging her path to becoming a nurse-anesthetist. Like the superior person of the *I Ching* who does not deviate from his or her purpose, Tow persevered firmly in her dream and her destiny until her goal to practice medicine manifested in its physical, earthly form and passion.

Conclusion

With benevolence Tow practiced a medicine rooted in healing principles, a practice nurtured by her early learning of Confucian and Taoist teachings. Through our reading of her dialogues in **Strange Kindness**, we not only observe, but also recreate with her a practice of benevolence that manifested as *Zhong,* faithfulness, and *Su,* forgiveness. We also participate in Tow's generosity of spirit, a generosity that creates **Strange Kindness** and aims to honor all the people who guided or aided her to fulfill her life's purpose on earth.

Harmony of Kindness and Strange: Reading *Strange Kindness* through the Lenses of Holistic, Western Medical Art and Poetry Therapy

a commentary by Stephen Rojcewicz

Chu Cho-Shin (Mabel S. Chu Tow), through the wholeness of her life, her practice as a nurse anesthetist and her writing as a poet, and the synthesis of her oral history is a superb example of the integration of science and art, the humanization of the healing profession, the harmony of western technology with the wisdom of traditional Chinese medicine, and the promise of poetry therapy.

A major pathology of modern times has been the barrier between science and the humanities, what C. P. Snow in 1956 called "The Two Cultures," hostile forces of science and the arts, facing mutual incomprehension and even contempt.[1] Such a barrier would have appeared as a monstrous aberration to the mind of someone steeped in traditional Chinese medicine and culture, as well as to western physicians of earlier centuries.

Despite the cleavage and rhetoric of the Two Cultures, the medical arts and poetry have been integrally linked for millennia. Physicians and healers have been inspired by poets, and have created great poetry and literature. The list of American physician poets, for example, includes William Carlos Williams (1883-1963), probably the greatest American physician poet to date; Oliver Wendell Holmes (1809-1894); Silas Weir Mitchell (1829-1914), a well-known neurologist and writer, and at one time, a critic of psychiatry for not being scientific enough; and contemporary doctors such as Rafael Campo and Jack Coulehan. Among British writers, John Keats (1795-1821) had been a medical student, although he never practiced medicine; and Oliver Goldsmith (1738-1774) was a physician. In the late eighteenth century, Erasmus Darwin, a physician and the grandfather of Charles Darwin, composed a two-volume poetic work, in decasyllabic rhymed couplets, on botany, with an emphasis on the medicinal value of plants; he was reputed to have polished his epic work riding in his carriage, between visits to his patients.[2] European physician writers include Francois Rabelais (1490-1553), Friedrich von Schiller (1759-1805), and Anton Chekhov (1860-1904).

Traditional Chinese medicine was steeped in the overall culture of this great civilization, where writings and practices integrated medical, artistic and literary skills, such as the *Yellow Emperor's Classic of Medicine* (*Hung Di Nei Jing*) in the Warring States Period (475 B.C. to 221 BCE), and the *Illustrated Manual of Acupuncture and Moxibustion Points on the Bronze Figure* written by Wang Wei Yi during the T'ang Dynasty in 1026. Wang Wei Yi accompanied his text with two life-size bronze figures that he had cast in order to standardize the acupuncture points.[3] Practitioners of Chinese traditional medicine were also intimately familiar with classics such as *Tao Te Ching* and *I Ching*. The doctors were experts in arts such as calligraphy; clients would choose a doctor by examining his calligraphy: an illustration of the people's acceptance of the intrinsic harmony of the arts and the sciences. Few Western physicians would be chosen on the basis of the penmanship of their prescriptions.

In both western and traditional Chinese medicine, poetry and the medical arts have enriched each other: through disciplined observation of concrete details, the study of basic biological phenomena (such as the importance of rhythm in heart function and in breathing), a mindful attentiveness to nature, a focus on sensory aspects, a search and examination for universal values, and an appreciation of harmony. In addition, the classics of Chinese civilization strengthen traditional Chinese medicine and can inspire the best of modern Western medical arts with a gratitude for the gift of healing, a sense of humility and reverence, and a fundamental compassionate response to the mystery of human suffering. The life and writings of Mabel Tow well illustrate these themes.

Strange Kindness and Poetry Therapy

Mabel Tow begins her oral history with what seems like an apology. Now that she is old, she states, she is responsible for her own nature; she continues that she has not yet honored "the strange kindness/ of my angels." She asks, "How can I honor/ my angels?"

Such an attitude of deference and humility is the beginning of a full appreciation of all the people who have influenced and helped her. The ensuing oral history is a tribute to these individuals, these angels who, in Taoist teaching, connect heaven and earth, and guide in providing balance to our lives. From the start, Tow's composing illustrates the poetry therapy process of life review in the elderly, in which individuals are encouraged to summarize their life stories through writing or dictation, returning to important memories and enhancing their current quality of life by finding overall meaning and purpose as well as creativity.[4]

We can speculate as to why Mabel Tow makes this apologetic statement that she has not honored her angels. The entire text of the oral history demonstrates that, indeed, her whole life has been an honoring of those who have guided her, from her dedication to her father's principles, to her diplomatic handling of the staff resentments against Dr. Ting, to her voyage to America and her subsequent career, to cite just a few examples. Her life-long attitudes and actions refute the premise, but Tow clearly states at the beginning of this work that she has not honored the strange kindness of her angels.

One answer to this paradox may come from the field of poetry therapy. Poetry therapy (or Bibliotherapy) is the intentional use of poetry and other forms of literature for healing and for personal growth. The defining characteristic of poetry therapy, as contrasted with other forms of therapy or of personal development is the central role of literature (a poem, song, play, movie, oral history, memoir, autobiography, work of fiction, etc.). In both clinical and developmental settings, poetry therapy is an interactive process with usually three essential components: the literature, the therapist or facilitator, and the client.[5]

Its practitioners can be therapists, physicians, nurses, psychologists, pastoral counselors, teachers, writers, librarians, etc. Poetry therapy can take place in clinical situations, for treatment of specific disorders and conditions, and can be practiced within individual psychotherapy, marital and family psychotherapy, and group psychotherapy formats. It is not limited to any one theoretical orientation, but can be used by trained therapists and facilitators who hold a variety of theoretical positions. As the late Arthur Learner, Ph.D., a distinguished California practitioner of poetry therapy, pointed out, poetry therapy is a "tool, not a school."[6] Poetry therapy also is applied in a developmental context, for enhancement of personal growth and insight.

Three major components comprise poetry therapy: a) the receptive/prescriptive mode; b) the expressive/creative mode; and c) the symbolic/ceremonial mode.[7] Using a group psychotherapy format, for example, the poetry therapist selects a poem or other form of written or spoken media to serve as a catalyst and to evoke feeling responses for discussion. In the expressive/creative mode, an already existing poem is chosen. The focus is on the person's reaction to the literature, not on literary merit per se. The symbolic/ceremonial mode emphasizes the power of rituals to validate an occurrence, promote change, and bring closure. This occurs naturally throughout medicine, psychotherapy and the life cycle, but poetry therapy makes explicit what is often implicit, and utilizes these events for therapeutic and developmental gain. An important example of the symbolic/ceremonial mode is encouraging the client to write a letter to an important person who is no longer available, detailing the patient's emotional reactions to that person or wishes to end an interpersonal conflict or misunderstanding.

What Mabel Tow has done is to take the recurrent themes of her life and put them in writing. She has created the literature, her autobiographical poem. Her entire life certainly honors the strange kindness of her angels; her oral history, however, honors her angels in a related but more intense way, a way that will persist long after she has died, and long after the memories pass away in those individuals who have personally known Mabel Tow. The first two stanzas of *Strange Kindness* can be seen as the beginning of both the expressive/creative mode and the symbolic/ceremonial mode of poetry therapy.

In addition, her oral history, once dictated or written down, becomes an additional catalyst for awareness and self-discovery. Tow refers frequently to the opening lines, refines the theme of honoring her angels, interacts with her memories, enriches the associations to angels and friends and to the healing arts, fine-tunes her understanding, attains additional insight, and ultimately honors her angels profoundly.

Melissa Ann Reed, in her *Introduction*, quotes a poem by Mabel Tow that illustrates this process:

> I think about my memories
> and this poem that will be
> forever like our friendship,
> always unfolding

The final lines of her oral history are thus a poem that symbolically fulfills the promise of the opening stanzas:

> Leaves wave slowly on their branch,
> Clouds flow around,
> Fragrant wind touches my face.
>   Oh, wind, could you touch my friends far away?
>   Give them my soft words?

Goals of Poetry Therapy

The goals of poetry therapy can be summarized below.[8] This list is not exhaustive, but it can be seen that many of these goals are fulfilled by Mabel Tow's oral history. The stated goals of poetry therapy are: a) to promote change, increase coping skills and improve adaptive functions, in order to work through underlying conflicts; b) to heighten participants' reality orientation; c) to enable participants to ventilate overpowering emotions and release tension; d) to encourage positive thinking and creative problem solving; e) to strengthen participants' communication skills, especially their willingness to listen carefully and to speak directly; f) to enhance participants' self-understanding and accuracy in self-perception; g) to encourage participants' awareness of personal relationships; h) to encourage participants' capacity to respond to vivid images and concepts, and the feelings aroused by them; i) to encourage or balance participants' creativity and self-expression, and their greater self-esteem; j) to help participants experience the liberating and nourishing qualities of harmony and beauty; k) to increase participants' spontaneity and capacity for playing with words and ideas; l) to help participants find new meaning through new ideas, insights, and/or information; and m) to help participants integrate the different aspects of the self for psychological wholeness.

Mabel Tow indicates that these goals are fulfilled not only through her life, but also through her writings. The poem in Section 17 compares the gradual unfolding of her feelings to moonlight emerging through branches:

> Moonlight shines
> through tree branches
> into my heart.

I don't like you
when you try to learn
my secret.

I love you
when you let me tell you
what I want to tell you.

By the end of her oral history, Tow has indeed told us what is in her heart. It is certainly true that a light that shines into her heart has enabled this accomplishment. This light, symbolized by moonlight in Section 17, gives rise to a partial self-revelation at that time. The full light of insight will come from writing her poems and dictating her oral history, and then reflecting on what she has written and experienced. The original poems, such as the one on moonlight, are catalysts that evoke feeling responses. The ultimate moonlight is the process of continuing to work on her oral history, and further reflecting on what she has produced. Through her writings, Tow has fulfilled the poetry therapy goals of enhancing self-understanding and accuracy in self-perception; awareness of personal relationships; helping to find new meaning through new ideas, insights, and/or information; and helping to integrate the different aspects of the self for psychological wholeness.

The Praying Mantis

One of Tow's central memories is the experience, at age nine, of saving a praying mantis from drowning; the insect then removes the wart from her thumb (Section 18). This episode reverberates with multiple allusions and meanings: reverence for all life, the importance of prayer, the tension between filial challenge and filial devotion, a foreshadowing of other people's saving of Tow's life, encouragement of others to experience freedom, the condition of the oneness of the universe (*tian ren he yi*), and the reciprocity of healing to cite just a few of the meanings.

I would like to use this memory as an example of the congruence between Tow's study of traditional Chinese medicine and the practice of poetry therapy. Tow's language, here as elsewhere, is poetic and imaginative. She describes her father as "a little out of breath" when returning from the pond with the mantis, and her father then describes the mantis in these words: "He's all wet now. / He can't pray." The use of language is telling. Why does her father have to be "out of breath"? What is the connection between the mantis being wet, and being unable to pray?

Traditional Chinese medicine often regards disease as arising from emotions interacting with external causes, or as arising from factors that have disturbed the harmony and balance of the whole energy system of the organism, disturbing both the physical body and the emotions.[9] Her father's being out of breath may signal this disturbance involving both the physical body and the emotions, especially because this is the first time that Tow has challenged her father. Her father is also using this occasion to teach Tow to be acutely observant of sensory qualities, and how they reflect the inner life: (the underlining in the following quote is mine)

> You see.
> Now observe.
> Two little legs are together.
> That's praying.
> You watch the mantis pray.

Shigehisa Kuriyama has compared the traditional Chinese medical model with the western model as enunciated by the ancient Greeks. He finds widely different perspectives in these medical models, expressed through language, touch, sight, breath, and identity. The western emphasis on anatomy and muscle is contrasted with the traditional Chinese focus on more sensory aspects: pulse, color, etc.[10] Dr. Chu, among many other things, is teaching his daughter to observe carefully, to focus on smell and tactile sensations in her diagnostic skills (an approach somewhat archaic in western medicine since the advent of CT scans and specialized X-rays), to use her observations to develop empathy for others and increased self-awareness, and to consider what the observed sensory qualities reveal of the inner life (e.g., the mantis is now praying). Tow, indeed, uses this episode to develop her skills of natural observation and to begin her own journey into self-knowledge.

These qualities of mindful attention, introspection, self-awareness, empathy, intuition and the beginnings of a psychological journey into self-knowledge are precisely the requirements needed for the development of poetry therapists and for the selection of the specific literature to be used in poetry therapy.[11] Tow's account of the Praying Mantis would itself make an excellent strategic choice of material to be used by facilitators for poetry therapy work in therapeutic and developmental settings.[12]

The Buddhist Prohibition

One episode in Tow's life that is difficult to understand is her father's prohibition on reading the Buddhist books. Dr. Chu had allowed his young daughter to accompany her mother, a Buddhist, to a Buddhist temple. He then takes Tow aside, and cautions her, "but do not read their books." She did not then understand why, and even toward the end of her life, she still wondered why (Section 6). It is a tribute to her love for truth that Tow cites this puzzling episode.

I would like to offer some speculations on this prohibition of reading the Buddhist books, from the standpoint of the possible convergence of traditional Chinese medicine and modern western medicine.

Norman Girardot, in his study of the symbols for chaos in early Taoism, contrasts the Taoist emphasis on chaos (*hun-tun*) with the fundamental values of other classical Chinese systems of thought, such as the Confucian emphasis on hieratic order, or the texts of Buddhist beliefs. Mythologically, in Taoism, chaos is the secret source of creation. The Taoist sage prefers to follow his inner urge and intuition rather than blindly to accept rigid order and authoritarianism, or to be limited to Buddhist scripture. Chaos (or perhaps strangeness), with its multiple and rich meanings, suggests the presence of a higher and more authentic order.[13] The spirit of Taoism has certainly influenced traditional Chinese medicine. Dr. Chu is preparing his daughter to rely on her own experience and intuition, even if her intuition and her life seem chaotic at times, rather than to follow any pre-set system. Dr. Chu is saying: "Don't rely solely on canonical texts; be open to the strange kindness of angels."

In addition, one of the fundamental precepts of Buddhism is that suffering exists. As a recent magazine article suggests, a strictly Buddhist context might lead to this conclusion: "Because sickness and death are inevitable, resisting them brings more misery, not less."[14]

Dr. Chu is perhaps telling his daughter to become a healer, despite the universality of suffering; to relieve pain, even if the relief is only temporary; and to treat sickness, despite the inevitability of death. I am reminded of the advice to doctors by a Greek physician in early Roman times, Aretaeus the Cappadocian, who composed treatises on the *Cure of Melancholy*, on *Madness*, and *Acute and Chronic Diseases*: "It is impossible, indeed, to make all the sick well, for a physician would thus be superior to a god; but the physician can produce respite from pain, intervals in diseases, and render them latent."[15]

The Harmony of Kindness and Strange

Traditional Chinese medicine identifies specific basic substances, such as qi (life-sustaining energy), jing (essence), blood, body fluids, and shen (mind or psyche). When the basic substances are in harmony, the individual will be fully alive and free of disease.[16] Tow's life and her oral history exemplify this spirit of harmony.

She has faced wartime, deprivations, cultural and geographical dislocation, professional loss, possible deportation, and the early death of her husband. Throughout her life, she has "chosen her own nature." She has opted for kindness, benevolence, harmony, healing. Her angels, in her well-chosen term, have been "strange": unexpected, from different cultures, coincidences (such as meeting Frank, and misunderstanding the sounds "Neuro" and "Uro"). Despite the strangeness of her angels, and the strangeness of all she had to face, Tow is like the Taoist garden in Lily Tsang's commentary: yin and yang in harmony. Tow overcomes or makes the most of her obstacles, accepts her suffering, and in her oral history, places her entire life in perspective. Her life and her writings provide a new synthesis, the harmony of western technological medicine with the wisdom of traditional Chinese medicine. Death and human suffering are issues that by their very nature are not amenable solely to technological solutions, such as medical procedures. These issues call for contemplation and reflection, for kindness in the face of strangeness. Death and suffering are what the French philosopher Gabriel Marcel has identified as "mysteries," issues that engage our full humanity, as opposed to simple "problems," which are technical questions that can be solved merely by technical means.[17]

Human illness, suffering and healing are true mysteries. A healer, such as Tow, responds to these mysteries by evoking the human mystery inside herself or himself. Strangeness is structured and transformed by kindness. Chaos gives rise to a higher order. Healing, as practiced by Tow and by all those who are physician-poets in their souls, combines the technical mastery of a medical problem with the response of the whole human being to the mystery of death and suffering. That response of the human healer, with empathy and scientific objectivity, concrete attention to detail, application to the individual situation, and openness to the universal, is truly poetry.[18] Tow's life and work is thus an integration of traditional Chinese medicine with modern western holistic medicine, an intersection of the humanities with the healing arts, a balance of empathy and intuition with scientific knowledge. Tow has overcome Snow's dichotomy of the Two Cultures of science and humanities, and has created a bridge between traditional Chinese and western medicine. *Strange Kindness* is a wonderful, inspiring example of holistic medicine, and of the promise of poetry therapy.

Endnotes

1. C. P. Snow, "The Two Cultures," in *New Statesman*, (October 6, 1956), pp. 413-14.

2. E. Darwin. *The Botanic Garden: a Poem in Two Parts*. London: J. Johnson, 1791.

3. W. Mao. "The Rise, Fall and Renaissance of Traditional Chinese Medicine," in *Acupuncture Today*, Volume 04, Issue 11, November, 2003.

4. S. Reiter, "Enhancing the Quality of Life for the Frail Elderly: Rx: the Poetic Prescription," *Journal of Long-Term Home Health Care*, 13 (1994), pp.12-19.

5. S. Reiter, "Poetry Therapy: Testimony on Capitol Hill," *Journal of Poetry Therapy*, 10 (1997), pp. 169-78.

6. A. Lerner, Ed. *Poetry in the Therapeutic Experience*. St. Louis: MMB Music, 1994.

7. N. Mazza. *Poetry Therapy: Interface of the Arts and Psychology*. Boca Raton, FL: St. Lucie Press, 1999.

8. S. Rojcewicz, "Medicine and Poetry: the State of the Art of Poetry Therapy," in *International Journal of Arts Medicine* 6, 2 (2000), pp. 4-9.

9. M. J. Parker, "Traditional Chinese Herbal Medicine," in D. Novey, Ed, *Clinician's Complete Reference to Complementary & Alternative Medicine* (St. Louis: Mosby, 2000) pp. 203-18.

10. S. Kuriyama. *The Expressiveness of the Body and the Divergence of Greek and Chinese Medicine*. Cambridge, MA: MIT Press, 1999.

11. K. Adams and S. Rojcewicz, "Mindfulness on the Journey Ahead," in G. Chavis and L. Weisberger, Eds., *The Healing Fountain: Poetry Therapy for Life's Journey* (St. Cloud, MN: North Star Press, 2003) pp. 7-35.

12. A. M. Hynes and M. Hynes-Berry. *Biblio/Poetry Therapy: the Interactive Process.* St. Cloud, MN: North Star Press, 1986.

13. N. Girardot. *Myth and Meaning in Early Taoism: the Theme of Chaos (Hun-Tun).* Berkeley: University of California Press, 1983.

14. K. Schulz, "Did Antidepressants Depress Japan?" in *The New York Times Magazine*, (August 22, 2004), p. 40.

15. Aretaeus. *The Extant Works of Aretaeus, the Cappadocian.* Edited and translated by F. Adams, (Boston: Longwood Press, 1958 [reprint of Sydenham Society Edition, London, 1856]) p. 222. Original work written circa 150 CE.

16. Parker, *op. cit.*, 204-5.

17. G. Marcel. *Being and Having*. New York: Harper and Row, 1965. Original work published 1935.

18. S. Rojcewicz, "*Puzzling Question* and the Poetry of Healing," in *Journal of Poetry Therapy,* 8 (1995), pp. 179-83.

Little Bamboo: A Five-Element Study of a Life Fully Lived

a commentary by David Naimon

I was asked to contribute to *Strange Kindness* because I am a westerner who practices a form of classical Chinese acupuncture called Five Element. In some respects my medical journey takes a trajectory opposite to that of Mabel. As a child I wanted to be a doctor. But as I moved through my pre-medical education, I became more enamored with other ways of approaching health and illness; first through naturopathic medicine, later with traditional Chinese medicine (TCM) and ultimately through Five Element acupuncture, the roots of which lie in the early shamanic traditions of Chinese medicine. I was never fortunate enough to meet Mabel Tow, but here I am offering some insights into her life's story from a classical Chinese perspective.

The Boundary Crosser: A Life with Unbound Feet

Imagine a Chinese shaman or "medicine woman" of old. She lived on the edge of the village. She was clearly not part of the town, but she was not entirely separate from it either. She was not a forest dweller, but she was a listener to the moods of the forest nonetheless. She was an inhabitant of that ambiguous zone where village fades and forest has not quite begun. If you could look down from above, from an eagle's vantage point, upon the daily movements of the townspeople, you would notice that their movements, day in and day out, stayed within a certain circumscribed pattern. Perhaps a morning spent in the fields, a trip to the market, a visit to a relative. The shaman's house was not approached on these quotidian journeys. Thoughts of the shaman would not inhabit the minds of the people at these times. When their lives were in balance, and their movements flowed with the rising and setting of the sun, with the seasons, and within society, the shaman was not part of their reality.

The shaman lived outside the habits of humans. Only when a villager's life tipped out of balance, from the culmination of poor lifestyle choices or from an unforeseen tragedy or illness, would a villager step outside his normal trajectory and visit the shaman. The illness itself literally called for changes to one's path. And one physically had to leave the comfortable patterns of one's daily rhythms to gain insight from someone, or some force larger than that provided from the everyday human cultural and social fabric.

The location of the shaman provided her this vantage point. The shaman became a barometer of the relationship between the community and the natural environment that sustained it. But she was not just a barometer. She was also a medium through which harmony could be reestablished between the individual and the community, and between the community and Nature. Unlike the townsperson, she often ventured forth into the wilderness, into landscapes unshaped by the human mind. Her tools were found here, deep within the forest. She unearthed medicines, harvesting roots and stems that otherwise lay hidden and unseen.

What relevance this has for Mabel Tow's story, you may wonder. The shaman lived on the edge of a village, in a transition zone. She placed herself physically in this position because her medicine, particularly her ability to restore balance, arose by living in liminal spaces, upon thresholds that defied easy categorization. Mabel's life unfolded in a similar manner, transcending category. Her life inhabited liminal spaces, and like the shaman, she sought knowledge that is only found by the crossing of thresholds.

From the very beginning, when Tow's father dressed her as a boy, he chose for Mabel an unusual life. "Make sure my Little Bamboo's feet are not bound." From this moment Mabel's role in the world would not be one easily defined. Her unbound feet were a statement that her voyage would cross boundaries, that her life would hold steady in the mystery of paradox. This life came with a cost however. Education and liberation separated her from her own family and from the community of women around her. But as her life path took form, it was clear that she was on a road with few travelers, a road that crossed the boundaries, not only of gender but of culture, religion, language and tradition as well. A woman unbound, she was a Christian from China, and a Chinese woman in America. She was a foreign navigator of American culture, yet a practitioner of western medicine whose life unfolded in a distinctly Taoist way: by the paradoxical principle of *wu wei*, action arising from non-action. A Mandarin speaker in an English world, and a gentle soul, who through yielding was able to overturn social convention, Mabel chose a life that unfolded according to its own dictates.

East Meets West: The Story of Dr. Ting and the Two Dishes

My teachers often mentioned the shaman as the epitome of classical Chinese approach to medicine, an approach entirely unlike the Western model, and likewise unlike many modern variants of Chinese medicine of the last half-century. Many of you are familiar with a common experience of visiting doctors. You have a pain you get a painkiller. You are depressed you get an anti-depressant. The western model has become a sophisticated tool to identify and remove symptoms. But where do these symptoms come from? A more holistic doctor might acknowledge the symptoms as the expression of a deeper imbalance within the human organism. But in classical Chinese approach, the origin of the symptom does not lie within the individual. It lies within the individual's relationship with Nature and, even in some cases, it is an expression of a community's imbalanced relationship with Nature. Thus, an acupuncture mentor warned me not to let my desire to alleviate suffering become an attempt to remove symptoms. If the practitioner merely treated the symptoms and made them go away, she would be ignoring the cause. And with the cause—an imbalance between the village, the country, the species—unattended to, the symptom would just manifest in someone else in the community. Thus the shaman could not be fully of the community she was with. She had to live in that interface. To hone her senses, to be able to diagnose with sounds, smells, colors and emotion.

Early in Mabel's life, she was trained in Classical Chinese Medicine, and we know that later in her life, she still remembered acupuncture points and their functions, as well as various Chinese herbal remedies for common ailments. The mystery lies in how Mabel's early exposure to Classical Chinese Medicine and how her upbringing in pre-Maoist China may have influenced her approach to medicine, to caretaking, to the art of living.

One of the main differences between a western medical approach and a Chinese one is that the former views events as a sequence of causes and effects, the latter, as unfolding pattern and process. Someone throws a rock at a window. Did the rock cause the window to break? No, they are two expressions of the same underlying process unfolding. They arose mutually as an expression of the rock thrower's inner state. Health, in its true sense, can only be restored, not by removing rocks, but by addressing the process within the rock thrower. A classical practitioner might observe a person's liver pain, the unusually early and harsh summer, an over-consumption of spicy foods, and the erosion of the river bank, where water was retrieved and consumed, as part of the same underlying pattern of imbalance.

The story of Dr. Ting and the two dishes exemplifies this approach of pattern and process perfectly. Nineteen of Dr. Ting's employees had forgotten the larger perspective. The nineteen voiced their grievance about Dr. Ting to Mabel. "We eat only two dishes," complained one. "Dr. Ting is off to enjoy himself," accused another. "While we have to suffer alone," concluded the first. "While Dr. Ting eats well in the U.S.," continued the second, "we wonder who else eats better than we do at home." These employees could only see the symptom, the two dishes, but not the larger picture of interconnectedness that Mabel so eloquently stated:

You eat only two dishes.
We staff eat the same two dishes.
I am sure Dr. Ting would be eating
the same way we do.
He is one of us.

You can see that everyone has trouble.
Patients cannot always pay for their rooms.
It isn't just you or us.
This isn't Dr. Ting's doing.
It is our country that is in trouble.
Don't you think we all would like to have peace?

No more war?
Because of war,
everyone has difficulty.
Let's remember our benefits
and Dr. Ting's care.

Here, Mabel contextualizes the complaints of the employees within the larger perspective of the status of the country as a whole. And she continues with one of the employees, pointing out that one's grievance may not be a grievance at all: "Your wife just had a baby in this hospital. She received complete care—did not pay a penny." After this, there were not nineteen employees speaking at once. Just the silent observation of the broader truth.

When a Name is Not Just a Name: The Virtue of Bamboo

The naming of Mabel as "Little Bamboo" was prescient. Her life unfolded much like the qualities of bamboo. *The bamboo that bends is stronger than the oak that resists.* Bamboo is a symbol of humility in China, but the qualities of bamboo are actually much more nuanced than this. Bamboo is often used as a prime example of the essence of the wood element in Five Element Theory.

Bamboo has three important qualities. It's empty, it's yielding and it's rooted. A person with a healthy wood energy is resilient, and able to adapt to unforeseen obstacles. Bamboo is a good example of this. It is "empty," or hollow, because it is not attached to the moment. In fact, in the moment it seems to yield to whichever way the wind is blowing. But despite this, it never is uprooted. It grows vigorously according to its inner plan.

Wind is the climactic factor associated with the wood element. It represents the unpredictable nature of life. Mabel's life was certainly full of windiness, opportunities to become frustrated and uprooted. Her imminent deportation, her nursing degree which initially would not be honored in the United States, her struggles with English and with American culture, and Frank's illness were just a few of these unforeseen obstacles. "If you don't think I should be an anesthetist, then just give me peace." Mabel could have lost hope, but instead she yielded to moments that refrained from providing answers. She waited for the way to open. And her "angels," the people who appeared fortuitously in her life to help her fulfill her heart's desire, redeemed her.

"I have strong feelings that anesthesia is my life's work." Being empty and yielding without being uprooted requires vision. Vision is also associated with the wood element. One of the two organs of the wood element, the liver, creates our vision for the future. In fact, the spirit that inhabits the liver, the spirit that the liver houses and nourishes, is the one that survives our death according to Chinese medicine. Thus the liver is planning for the ultimate demise of our physical body. Appropriately the liver is associated with the eyes. Mabel's life unfolded according to her inner vision.

Equally important to a healthy wood element is appropriate timing and decisiveness. This is the role of the gallbladder, the other wood organ, which executes the plan and vision of the liver. This occurs, even on the most basic level in our bodies. For instance, the liver plans for the digestion of our future meals by creating bile in advance of them. The gallbladder holds the bile, and squirts it on the food as it passes by in the small intestine. Thus timing and decisiveness is essential for the gallbladder to be successful. "Though peace came to me, I was never satisfied. What could I do to change my circumstance?" Paradoxically, despite bamboo's seemingly endless bending, it also springs back, and resumes its chosen path at the first opportunity.

"Leaves wave slowly on their branch." Mabel's poem exemplifies the energy of the wood element that she so wonderfully brought into the world. "Clouds flow around." When the wood element is healthy, there is a sense of "smooth flow" or benevolence. A life guided by angels. "Fragrant wind touches my face." Mabel had befriended the obstacles in her life, as opportunities, as friends. "Oh wind, could you touch my friends far away? Give them my soft words?" And like the soft seedling that pushes upward in springtime, through the hardest and coldest ground, it is Mabel's very softness that allowed her to become her life's dream.

Heart-mind Biopoetics and Tow's Moon Door

a commentary by Melissa Ann Reed

Before birth
in semiotic fluid bearing
the language and lights
of the universe,
our infant heads unfurl
up, out of our hearts,
flower buds from calyx shields.

Heart cells create,
clothe the third eye,
which will beat open
each one's unique insight,
psyche's way to shape
bios in synergy
with rhyme, reason,
and rhythms of heart.

Heart cells create,
clothe the ears,
which will beat open
our listening with ear of heart,
with attunement
to nature's subtle sounds—
the wind made by rabbit's feet
through silken grass.

So Chinese shamans saw
with their third eyes
our subtle, light bodies—
the movement of light
between heart, ears, third eye,
and Baihui crowning our heads,
that sacred, empty space,
Beginner's Mind
where all meridians meet,
where heaven, earth, and child
may one another greet.*

*First published in the *Empty Vessel*, Summer 2004.

"Close your eyes. . . . See the upper half of your body in the sky, the lower half rooted in the earth." So begins Master Zhongxian Wu's shamanic qigong class. "Visualize yourself in a very green forest. Notice the large leaves on the trees." So begins Madame Liu He's water-fire mudra of Jade Leaves qigong. "Think of a pleasant image." So begins surgery at the nurse-anesthetist's suggestion. These practices aim to engage the agent of healing within us by drawing upon our capacities to imagine, to think with images. Images—visual, auditory, kinesthetic—comprise an unconditional language, a kind of prenatal umbilical cord, connecting us with the unconditional world of spiritual truth. Images, emergent from heart-mind in connection with the pulse of the life-force, remind us of our intrinsic connection with the universe, the biosphere, the nonhuman world, the stardust in our bones, and the mind-body-spirit triad of our humanity. Biopoetics is the study of these connections. A term first conceived by the scholar of speech-communication, Kenneth Burke, biopoetics refers to bios, the body's observed capacity to think in images, and poetics, the psyche's observed capacity to shape relationships with bios to make meaning through symbols or symbolic action.[1] Accordingly, biopoetics primarily studies how the symbolic action of speech-interpretation creates (or fails to create) a life-giving relationship between bios and the faculty of imagination. However, not all symbolic actions are verbal. This commentary brings the template of biopoetics to bear upon our understanding of three ways to shape relationships with bios through primarily nonverbal symbolic action: the medical art of qigong, the medical art of inducing hypnosis with anesthesia, and Tow's art of awakening that felt-sense of wonder and awe so crucial to the free flow of life's energy. All three of these ways are at work as Tow shapes the moon door, the mending dialogue of *Strange Kindness*.

The Template of Biopoetics

Jungian analyst, Marion Woodman, shares the story of one of Carl Gustav Jung's patients, whose repressed feelings impaired his kidney function.[2] This patient first dreamed of a frozen river, later learning through medical diagnosis that his kidneys were becoming dysfunctional. The dream was the subtle, light body's metaphorical language, communicating the dreamer's physical situation and illuminating the spiritual meaning. Emergent from imagination or the body's capacity to think in images and the psyche's capacity to make symbolic meaning with those images, the dream also expressed the dreamer's motive of moral constraint against harm—the motive for creating a mending dialogue between the suffering body and healing agent within him. Such a mending dialogue would spring from the dream's metaphor, taking the shape of warming the frozen river, releasing the patient's laughter and tears, freeing his capacity for song and care, "the holiness of the heart's affections,"[3] all of which, when frozen, exert a modifying influence upon the body's capacity to function as a biological organism. In this case then, the diagnostic dream encodes the treatment: Release the patient's affect. His capacity to form a relationship with the life of his feelings will correct the course of illness, underlying and causing the symptoms of his kidney disease.

Though Jung did not know why an insufficient feeling life can break down a kidney, he intuited that the connection involved the psyche or the subtle, light body. Modern science now provides empirical understanding. Neuropeptide receivers receive images, and these images either negatively or positively affect the body's chemistry.[4] A person holding negative, restrictive images may release those old images, becoming open to receive new, positive images, thus changing cell metabolism and increasing immunoglobin-A needed for general health and a strong immune system.

That said, removal of a negative, restricting image is not always easy. A master "surgeon," the Elizabethan poet and dramatist, Shakespeare, attempts such a removal through the creative movement of *Sonnet 15*:

> When I consider every thing that grows
> Holds in perfection but a little moment,
> That this huge stage presenteth nought but shows
> Whereon the stars in secret influence comment;
> When I perceive that men as plants increase,
> Cheered and checked even by the selfsame sky,
> Vaunt in their youthful sap, at height decrease,
> And wear their brave state out of memory:
> Then the conceit of this inconstant stay
> Sets you most rich in youth before my sight,
> Where wasteful Time debateth with Decay
> To change your day of youth to sullied night,
> And all in war with Time for love of you,
> As he takes from you, I ingraft you new.[5]

The poet invites the reader to share in his empathic identification with both suffering person and beloved agent of healing. The one has no choice but to suffer entropy, depicted as an excruciating debate between wasteful Time and Decay. The other has a choice and chooses to reverse time and entropy through grace—through engrafting the suffering being to another kind of tree, one new in every moment. The image evoked is one of divine compassion never abandoning, but rather continually creating us anew.

This image of a real and viable, though often invisible phenomenon may remind us of the ancient Celtic tree of life, the one half green, the other half burning from its roots to its tip. There Spring and Autumn, sowing and reaping, both meet at one time. This image may also remind us of a dramatic scene under the microscope, the scene of old cells dying beside new cells being born, all in such a way that the whole life-force is never lost, is always, through natural selection, bringing something new into being. Once we receive a felt-sense that we are an integral part of this whole action, we may release the negative, restricting image in the body and hold the positive image of renewed life.

This positive image, often called genuine hope, engages the soul's animation or radiance. Radiance forms a new bridge of wholeness, a greater connection with the life-force than the one previously experienced.

We may also observe the divine interacting with a dislocated or imbalanced nature to create a mending dialogue between the suffering body and agent of healing within each creature. Through their consanguinity, the young student of classical Chinese medicine, Chu, Cho-Shin, and the distressed praying mantis meet in Dr. Chu's garden. Cho-Shin's awe and her empathic identification with the mantis initiate their mending dialogue, their greater connection to nature and to the Whole. Their mending dialogue involves two prayers of agency. Cho-Shin's active prayer magnifies and focuses the sun's fire to evaporate the excessive water in which the mantis could drown. The mantis's prayer of embodied stillness, after it receives the nutrition provided by Cho-Shin's wart, nourishes the spirit.

The Embodied Stillness of Qigong

Tow's story reveals what David Abrams calls the "animate intelligence" throughout the biosphere.[6] Her story reveals how the praying mantis as suffering body recognized her healing gifts: her moral constraint against its harm in a near-death condition, her natural compassion, and her heightened condition of wonder, which opens the heart to release vital energy to flow freely. Her story also reveals how the mantis as patient or agent of healing became her spirit guide, transmitting to her all the virtues of embodied stillness. From the praying mantis, she experienced not only the still point of vision outside the external world and ego-consciousness, enabling her to recognize the flow and the direction of the divine intervening in earthly events, but also the deep restfulness, which restores at-onement with the life-force. She experienced the consanguinity between her and all of nature, the necessity of removing excess, which restricts creative flow, and the natural balance achieved when an excess serves to fill a deficiency. She learned that these conditions, working together, create an awe-inspiring harmony, one that reverses time and entropy.

Embodied stillness, according to the ***Dictionary of Insect Totems***, is the power that the praying mantis bestowed upon ancient Chinese shamans, who shaped the first meditative practice of stillness in motion called qigong. Qigong indeed invites the practitioner to quiet the mind by bringing consciousness within and by observing the inner landscape with the inner eye. Such observation generates awareness of the spiritual energy within one's being and the universe. Qigong practice then teaches the practitioner to merge with the lights of the universe, to use particular images to open the heart to the life-force, and to encourage the movement of this force along specific pathways known to strengthen and empower it through various organs and systems of the body. To improve qi and blood circulation, qigong releases the subtle, light body from restrictions that cause entropy. Within the subtle, light body, conscious telepathic communication is possible.[7] Within the subtle, light body, the psyche will be at home after death.[8]

As spirit-guide, the praying mantis initiated Tow to her career path and focused her to learn the healing art of qigong, an art that would later support her western medical art of inducing hypnosis and administering anesthesia. She would spend much of her later life tending patients under anesthesia who, like the praying mantis, would be in a near-death condition. Crucial to their care would be her keen observation.

Dramatizing how insect and child became agents of one another's healing through patience, this whole event not only initiated Tow to the form of her future practice, but it affirmed her life-purpose to be a physician, a healer of life in classical Chinese medicine's true sense of the word. Her final act of healing in this instance, the act of liberating the mantis, completely fulfilled the two major purposes of qigong: 1) to engage the condition of freedom that life's energy needs in order to flow effortlessly and 2) to increase the life-force as a gift to the spirit.

The Biopoetics of Increasing the Life Force as Gift to the Spirit

Qigong represents a variety of symbolic acts, which embody stillness to shape bios. The psyche directs each act of meditation, using particular images and movements to quiet the mind and to direct the energy of stillness to balance and to harmonize yin and yang. One such act is that of making and holding the *Pure Yang Mudra*. The *Pure Yang Mudra*, according to Master Zhongxian Wu, originated among Mt. Emei sages, whose shamanic qigong art stemmed from *I Ching* science. Made by both hands forming a tiny globe when little and middle fingers and thumbs lightly touch, while ring and index fingers remain open, this mudra embodies the closed and open lines of the *I Ching* hexagram 65 and the symbolic action of water (yin) and fire (yang) "rooting into one another through wood."[9] Embodiment of this symbolic action aims to evoke a particular five-element interaction first observed in nature: a natural, recurring interaction that Tow observed that day in her father's garden, when she held out the wood stick, perhaps bamboo, upon which the praying mantis could perch and pray, while fire and water rooted into one another to increase the life force.

This interaction was later described by Werner Zimmermann, who observed how rolling pebbles emit sparks under water, how water expands, and how the stones form the riverbed to become the river's "bread." This phenomenon implied for him that, if an oxide can be created in water by a ray of flame, like the union between oxygen and stone, then oxide-water can also be created.[10]

Wu expresses the symbolic action of the *Pure Yang Mudra* this way:

> . . . water represents "Jing" (essence) the mother-substance. Fire represents qi, the father-substance. The "marriage" is managed by the "flame" (mind). The result is that the life-force and vital energy grow, and the mudra is the bread of the "Shen" (spirit).[11]

In biopoetic terms, the qigong practitioner embodies the deep rest of stillness, sometimes called *patience*. We may experience such stillness embodied by the pine tree or the great sequoia or the forest of giant redwoods in California. Such stillness slows the breath and the heartbeat, connecting us with the generative life force. Then, by directing that life force through the *Pure Yang Mudra*, the qigong practitioner becomes the creatrix of fire and water energies, as well as the praying one, who marries these energies, permitting their frequencies of light to coalesce into a mending dialogue to benefit the spirit.

The agency marrying the frequencies of fire and water is that of imagination. Imagination is our "utmost conceptual power," claims the philosopher of aesthetics, Suzanne K. Langer.[12] Imagination is "rooted in the heart's spiritual truth," claims the Jungian analyst, Evangeline Kane.[13] Imagination integrates mind, body, and spirit according to the *Yellow Emperor's Classic of Medicine*. Accordingly, the passion of patience and the spirit of truth combine within the agent of healing, the qigong practitioner, to engage imagination. Imagination then acts like a magnifying glass to intensify and to focus the light of fire and the light of water until they coalesce into a new frequency of light. Such an act also reverses time and entropy.

The concept of growing and directing vital energy by means of imagination or benevolent intention emerged, writes Adeline Yen Mah, from the classical Chinese physician's perception of healing as "a psycho-physiological force connected to the flow of breath, blood and inner thoughts."[14] This perception is not foreign to Western perceptions of healing, if we consider Asclepius's poetic healing practice of dream incubation and interpretation[15] and the writings of Hippocrates and Galen.[16] This perception is indeed not foreign to the mind of the actor, poet, and theatre artist, William Shakespeare.[17]

Writing on Shakespeare's imagery and what it tells us, Caroline Spurgeon finds that this actor-poet's

> Sensitive understanding of the influence of mind on body is what, however, puts him nearest to modern expert opinion, and this is as marked in his early as later work. Thus the whole story of the cause and development of madness in a brain over-strained with exasperation and anguish is sketched in *The Comedy of Errors*, fifteen years before the full portrait of it is drawn in *King Lear*.[18]

Composing with a sensitive understanding of the influence of mind on body, Shakespeare eschewed the medieval medical chant of *cogita mori*, meaning *think on death*, and offered a radically different healing visualization in his **Sonnet 146**: *Within be fed, without be rich no more: /So shalt thou feed on death, that feeds o men, /And death once dead, there's no more dying then.*[19]

Finally, the classical Chinese physician's perception of healing as a psycho-physiological force corresponds well with the psychobiology of gene expression theorized by the Jungian analyst and physician of medical hypnosis, Ernest L. Rossi.[20]

Medical Hypnosis and the Healing Imagination

Biopoetics regards the practice of medical hypnosis developed by Milton H. Erickson as still another way in which the symbolic action of psyche shapes relationship with bios. Writing about his practice, Erickson stressed how therapeutic hypnosis engages the subject as an agent of healing:

> . . . therapy results from an inner re-synthesis of the patient's behavior achieved by the patient himself. By such indirect suggestion the patient is enabled to go through those difficult inner processes of disorganization, reorganization, reassociating, and projecting of inner real experience to meet the requirements of the suggestion and thus the induced anaesthesia becomes a part of his experiential life instead of a simple, superficial response . . . . [21]

Erickson found this process of catalyzing the agent of healing within the subject a function of the interpersonal relationship between subject and hypnotist, a relationship that must adapt to the different personality needs of each subject.[22] Erickson also stressed the importance of the hypnotist's healing purpose to support the subject's intrinsic self-worth, well-being, and capacity for wholeness, instructing his subjects to form a positive relationship with their unconscious minds, "to let nothing disturb them, to enjoy their trance state . . . and full confidence in themselves, their situation, and their ability to meet adequately and well any problem or task that may be presented to them."[23]

We may well ask what the trance condition is. Is trance like that deep rest found in meditation? In qigong practice? Or is trance altogether different? Rossi's research suggests that trance is a deep, natural rest, during which subjects may also be enchanted or entranced by the numinous.[24]

After inducing trance, Erickson encouraged the subject's own psyche to grow and to shape authentic, meaningful, and healing relationships with bios. Erickson's practice established that imagery

> . . . permits the subject to utilize his actual capabilities without being hampered by an adjustment to non-essential externalities. This has been found true with experienced subjects as well as naïve subjects, and in the whole range of imagery from visual to kinesthetic.[25]

For instance, Erickson guided a patient, who was disturbed by her childhood learning of *The Ugly Duckling* story, to work with her negative images of the story as well as with new, positive images discovered outside the story, until she could shape a new, conscious relationship with the story, one supporting a positive self image.[26]

Erickson's work impacted the study and practice of Mind-Body Medicine, the use of hypnosis prior childbirth, and the nurse-anesthetist's use of suggestive technique prior surgery. Suggestive technique engages the patient's imagination for various purposes. According to the psychiatrist, Gerald Epstein, the function of imagination "is to act as an inner light, one that turns our attention toward the realm of the holy and to reverse time and entropy" such that our being becomes *negentropic*.[27] Suggestive technique also aims to use the patient's own mental imagery and capacity to be entranced by the numinous to reframe the heightened condition of fear before surgery into a heightened condition of wonder. This transformation relies upon the unconditional language of imagery to transport the subtle, light body into that matrix deeper than life and death, where all merges with the numinous light of the deepest kindness we can know.

A patient's positive mental and calm emotional condition prior surgery definitely can affect the success of surgery, according to cardiologist and surgeon, Dr. Hesham Zaki. Zaki's practice in Cairo, Egypt consists of caring for three patients at a time, offering them pre-surgical counseling and prayer "to build our faith," surgical intervention, and post-surgical nursing care. Zaki also teaches surgical nursing care and researches the underlying psychological problems of obesity and cardiac disease. He appreciates participating in all facets of medicine. "Patients whose faith was greater than mine definitely improved my surgical skills."[28]

Zaki's observation affirms the nurse-anesthetist or anesthesiologist, whose use of suggestive technique, at best, aims to guide the patient into a positive mental and peaceful emotional condition, one harmonizing with and aiding the surgeon's attitude and skill. Finally, "the nurse-anesthetist's skills can definitely affect a patient's recovery from surgery," shared Ladan Eshkevari, a nurse-anesthetist, physician of Traditional Chinese Medicine, and faculty member of Georgetown University's Nurse-Anesthetist Program.[29]

Examples of how patients have co-created health through imagery abound in Epstein's book, *Healing Visualizations*. His visualizations include meditations for mending bone fractures, correcting cardiac arrhythmia, correcting lack of version or rotating a fetus, and preparing for and recovering from surgery.[30]

Tow's Art of Awakening Wonder

"Think of a pleasant image." So begins surgery at the nurse-anesthetist's suggestion. Yet, how little time there is between the image that comes to mind and that fall into a deep sleep near death's door. So much depends upon the patient's inner resources. At the same time, so much depends upon how the nurse-anesthetist holds the sacred surgical space. A disciplined and exceptional degree of inner stillness transmits, entrains the cells of a patient and those of a surgical team, offering all a greater connection with the life force. A natural gift of heightened wonder may also transmit to open and to transport others into this same condition, wherein life's energy may freely flow. Tow impressed me with these gifts and skills, as she must have impressed all the patients and surgeons with whom she worked.

Wonder and awe are emotions evoked by heightened, deeply meaningful spiritual experiences, as may be had by realizing the unique, unrepeatable configuration of each snowflake or the agent of healing within a praying mantis.

The German scholar, Rudolph Otto, called such experiences *numinous*. Numinous and novel experiences may evoke unusually strong gene expression, brain plasticity, and mind-body healing at an unconscious level, according to Ernest L. Rossi. Rossi has developed a theoretical framework, integrating neuroscience and genetic research to provide the basis for studying the *Novelty-Numinosum-Neurogenesis Effect* with current neuroscience methods of brain imaging and DNA micro-array technology.[31] Perhaps future research will explore the impact of suggestive technique prior surgery at the genetic level.

Rossi also affirms how "replaying numinous dramas of healing that engage deep emotions, over and over, with many creative variations, allows a natural Darwinian process of variation and selection to take place on all levels, from mind to gene."[32] Mabel Tow replayed the Self-overheard dialogues of her life "many times." She told her story many times to many different sorts of people, some of whom she later regarded her angels. How well she must have understood the truth that every recall is a reframe, a creative opportunity to re-associate, reorganize and re-synthesize the meaning of the choices that "gave her today." How well her self-induced anesthesia must have become a part of her experiential life. The recipient of her last version, I would care to suggest, however, that this synthesis was not only a creative reframe to effect further self-healing, but also a gift to the spirit who engaged her wonder—a gift that would continue to grow the life force.

Tow's Moon Door

As Lily Tsang writes, the moon symbolizes for many Chinese "reunion, completeness, and awakened spirit," a doorway into the garden created by natural law. Could these symbolic associations give special meaning to the old Chinese proverb: *A book is a garden carried in the pocket*? Could Tow's book be her moon door, through which she and others may enter a beautiful garden? A garden like that most beautiful one, to which Wonderland's Alice longed to be admitted? Does Tow's story, like the moon door, create a special condition of reunion, completeness, and awakened spirit? Does her story, like the moon, create the conditions through which Kuan Yin and compassion can be born?

For Tow, who shared with me that she frequently conversed with the moon, this entity, reflecting soft light, represented "the spirit of freedom between listener and speaker." Representing the spirit of freedom, the moon was Tow's portal, permitting her free rite of passage back to her father's garden, the site of her early, life-shaping experiences. Furthermore, "the spirit of freedom" represented for her not only the spirit necessary for the effortless flow of life's energy, but also the spirit necessary to increase the life force—the spirit honored by her father's lesson, concerning how to create the mending dialogue between her and the praying mantis. The moon, then, returns Tow to the blessing of the mantis and the *pure yang mudra*--returns her to the time when, holding a stick of wood, she became creatrix of fire descending and water rising through wood, each rooting into the other to grow the life force as a gift to the spirit.

The gift of new life force yielded an amazing healing for both child and mantis. Moreover, the gift of new life force does not heal only once in one, particular circumstance. Wang, Xi Zhu's calligraphy, for example, increases the life force, and his gift to the spirit continues to transmit extraordinary life-energy to this very day! His numinous images, like Shakespeare's, reverse time and entropy.

Sensing the new life force transmitted through Tow's story and the aim and character from which it arises, I wonder further how such a speech-act "honors the strange kindness of her angels"? A clue exists in her poem, honoring the spirit of freedom between moon and poet, listener and speaker. To the moonlight, shining through tree branches into her heart, Tow writes, "I don't like you/ when you try to learn /my secret." Honor, like life-energy, needs to flow freely between people and does so when each regards the sanctity of the other's noble heart. Regarding the sanctity of the noble human heart was germaine to Tow's practice of inducing hypnosis and anesthesia. Just as the mystery of surgery was to be veiled from patients, their sacred, often unspoken images offered up by imagination prior surgery were to remain secrets.

Rossi stresses in *The Psychobiology of Gene Expression* and other articles how the practice of hypnosis respects the privacy of the client, how the client's inner discourse need not be shared, may be held in silence, never disclosed to the therapist. Conversely, Tow's angels, like good hypnotherapists, must have regarded the sanctity of her heart-mind, respecting, but not trying to learn her secrets.

We may ask further what this sanctity meant for Tow. From the Judeo-Christian wisdom tradition that Tow accepted, we read that God writes an inscrutable, not-to-be fathomed word of love within each of our hearts. Within each heart, God plants a different sacred text, and each sacred text will unfold like a tiny seed in God's good hand. These secrets, these not-to-be-fathomed words of love, function "to fabricate unknownness" according to the poet E. E. Cummings.[33] Unknownness, both unpredictable and whimsical, form the numinousity that opens our hearts and engages our imaginations, our connections with the light of unconditional love. The secret and sacred texts, written within each of her angels' hearts, are what Tow respects and aims to honor.

Time and again we observe her renouncing her will and accepting, even appreciating the kindness of her angels and the fabric of their unknownness, the faces of their strangeness that only God can know. For instance, Dr. Ting's gift was not to be resisted without harm to the flow of life, harm toward Ting's gesture of benevolence and gratitude. Therefore, Tow renounced her wish to see her beloved brother and accepted a larger dream for her life. "I couldn't say any more about my brother."

Similarly, she resisted mentioning to Father Reese her Buddhist practice, respecting the sacred cow, since her will would have wounded him. She chose rather to appreciate both what she could not understand, his strangeness, and what she could understand, the tender gravity of his kindness.

And when asserting her opinion could block the dance of kindness, she defers to the dance, conceding that two very different ways of tinseling a Christmas tree are "ok," since "each may be enjoyed in its own way." Does this speech-act within a particular scene, a scene celebrating the incarnation of divine love through nature, encompass how Tow approached integrating Chinese with western medicine, accepting the best from each way?

"Do I please myself or my father? That was my life-long question," Tow confided to me. When nearly deported from the U.S., however, she had to learn to release her father's vision for her life, only to receive several years later a profound affirmation of that vision from both Dr. Pender and her antagonist, Dr. Ridley. Plato taught that following one's bliss is fraught with self-renunciation; Tow teaches us that the path of our bliss is also fraught with strange kindness.

Endnotes

1. See Kenneth Burke. "Biology, Psychology, Words," in *Dramatism and Development*. Barre, Massachusetts: Clark UP, 1972. Lee Roloff. *Biopoetics: Energy of Language*. Oregon Friends of Jung Lectures, 1996.

2. Marion Woodman. *Sitting by the Well:* **Twelve Lectures**. Boulder, CO: Sounds True, 1998.

3. See John Keats. "Letter to Benjamin Bailey," in *Selected Poems and Letters*. Ed. Douglas Bush. Boston, MA: Houghton Mifflin, 1959.

4. See the research of James Pennebaker and Candace Pert.

5. William Shakespeare. "Sonnet 15," in *The Art of Shakespeare's Sonnets*. Ed. Helen Vendler. Cambridge: Harvard UP, 1997.

6. See David Abrams. *The Spell of the Sensuous*. NY: Pantheon Books, 1996.

7. Woodman, *Sitting by the Well*.

8. See Barbara Hanna. "The Unconscious Prepares for Death," in *Encounters with the Soul: Active Imagination*. Boston, MA: Sigo Press, 1981.

9. Zhongxian Wu. "Seeking the Roots of Classical Qigong: Exploring the Original Meaning of the Pure Yang Mudra," in *The Empty Vessel*, Winter 2003.

10. See Walter Zimmermann. "Fire under Water," in *The Water Wizard: The Extraordinary Properties of Natural Water*. Ed., Trans., Callum Coats. Bath: Gateway Books, 1998.

11. Wu, "Seeking the Roots of Classical Qigong."

12. Suzanne Langer. *Feeling and Form*. New York: Charles Scribner's Sons, 1953.

13. See Evangeline Kane. *Imagination and the Healing Process*. Boston, MA: Sigo Press, 1989.

14. See Adeline Yen Mah. *Watching the Tree*. New York: Broadway Books, 2001.

15. See Hymie Gordon. *The Cult of Asklepios*. Lecture 16, 1991. *History, Health, and Disease, Mayo Medical Association Lecture Series*.

16. See Hymie Gordon. *The School of Hippocrates*. Lecture 17, 1991. *Hellenism and the Alexandrian School of Medicine*. Lecture 18, 1991. *Galen and Medicine in Imperial Rome*. Lecture 20, 1991.

17. See Hymie Gordon. *Society and Medicine in Shakespeare's England*. Lecture 32, 1992. *Medical Beliefs and Practices in the Works of Shakespeare and His Contemporaries*. Lecture 33, 1992. David Hoeniger. *Medicine and Shakespeare in the English Renaissance*. Newark, NJ: University of Delaware Press, 1992. Edward Edinger.

The Psyche on Stage. Toronto: Inner City Books, 2001.

18. Caroline Spurgeon. *Shakespeare's Imagery and What it Tells Us.* Cambridge: Cambridge University Press, 1952.

19. Shakespeare, "Sonnet 146," in *The Art of Shakespeare's Sonnets.* Cambridge: Harvard University Press, 1997.

20. Ernest Rossi. *The Psychobiology of Gene Expression: Neuroscience and Neurogenesis in Hypnosis and the Healing Arts.* NY: W. W. Norton & Company, 2002.

21. Milton Erickson. "Hypnotic Therapy," in *The Collected Papers of Milton Erickson on Hypnosis.* Volume 1. *The Nature of Hypnosis and Suggestion.* Ed. Ernest Rossi. New York: Irvington, 1964/1980.

22. Milton Erickson. "Hypnosis in Medicine," in *The Collected Papers of Milton Erickson.* Volume 4. Ed. Ernest Rossi. New York: Brunner/Mazel, 1980.

23. Erickson, "Hypnosis in Medicine."

24. Rossi, *The Psychobiology of Gene Expression.*

25. Milton Erickson. "Deep Hypnosis and its Induction," in *Advanced Techniques of Hypnosis and Therapy.* Ed. Jay Haley. Orlando, FL: Grune & Stratton, 1967.

26. Erickson, "The Ugly Duckling: Transforming Self Image," in *The Collected Papers of Milton Erickson.* Volume 4.

27. Gerald Epstein, "Mental Imagery: The Language of Spirit in Mind-Body Medicine," in *Advances,* Volume 20, Number 3, Fall 2004.

28. Interview with Dr. Hesham Zaki, visiting cardiologist to Mayo Medical Community, July 1999.

29. Interview with Ladan Eshkevari, April 2004.

30. Gerald Epstein. *Healing Visualizations: Creating Health Through Imagery.* NY: Bantam, 2000.

31. Ernest Rossi, "Stress-Induced Alternative Gene Splicing in Mind-Body Medicine," in *Advances,* Volume 20, Issue 2, Summer 2004.

32. Ernest Rossi, "Sacred Spaces and Places in Healing Dreams: Gene Expression and Brain Growth Rehabilitation," in *Psychological Perspectives* 47, 1 (Los Angeles: C. G. Jung Institute, 2004) p. 61.

33. E. E. Cummings. *Complete Poems.* NY: W. W. Norton & Company, 1962.

Mabel Cho-Shin Tow

a commentary by Vay Liang W. (Bill) Go

Strange Kindness is the true-life story of Mabel Cho-Shin Tow. She ably bridged the East and the West, leaving her footprints everywhere and touching so many lives along the way. Her story spanned from pre-post-revolutionary China in Hankou City, Hu-Bei Province in 1914 to Shanghai in the 1940's and to her subsequent move to Rochester, Minnesota in 1949 until her death on November 1, 1999. She was one of the few early Chinese residents in Rochester, Minnesota, whose faith and tradition bridged Confucianism and Anglicanism and who was able to blend East and West cultural and traditional values in her life and in the medical practices of her profession. Over the years, Mrs. Tow became the adopted grandmother of the Rochester Chinese community and was a great role model who taught Chinese language, culture, and tradition. She also contributed significantly to community services and was recognized with the Rochester Golden Deed Award.

Mrs. Tow was also a great storyteller, and she started to reflect on her own life when we moved her to Charter House in 1988. She spoke often of her angels, the people who guided and helped her throughout her journey from the East to the West. Her angels were all great mentors, just like herself, always generous in giving guidance and nurturing her friendships, and so caring and loving to her lifelong friends.

Mrs. Tow always said that strong relationships are bidirectional and that it was always better to give than to receive. Along the way, she has been a great mentor to all of us, advising us on life, love, giving and caring, and God. In her own words, she would proudly say to us in her poem:

> Leaves wave slowly on their branch,
> Clouds flow around,
> Fragrant wind touches my face.
> Oh, wind, could you touch my friends far away?
> Give them my soft words?

ABOUT THE CONTRIBUTORS

Vay Liang W. (Bill) Go is Distinguished Professor of Medicine at David Geffen School of Medicine in Los Angles, California, Editor-in-Chief of *Pancreas*, and Tow's close family friend and guardian.

Charles Liu was born in Hong Kong in 1939 and learned Taoist Healing Arts and Chinese Medicine as a result of suffering from poor health during childhood. He studied electrical engineering at Boston's Northeastern University, subsequently completing a Master of Science degree at MIT. While working for IBM, Liu completed a doctorate with University of Minnesota faculty. Following early retirement from IBM, he began a second career as a Health Educator. He practiced Tuina (Acupressure) Message with Integrative Therapies at Assisi Heights and taught Tai Chi and Qigong in Rochester, Minnesota.

David Naimon is a naturopathic physician, a board certified Chinese herbalist, and licensed acupuncturist. He received his doctorate in Naturopathy and his Masters of Science in Oriental Medicine at the National College of Naturopathic Medicine. He later completed a three-year apprenticeship in Five-Element acupuncture. He currently practices in Portland, Oregon and hosts a weekly radio talk show called *Healthwatch*.

Melissa Ann Reed teaches English Literature and Theatre Arts for the International Baccalaureate Program at KDU Smart School in Malaysia. She completed doctoral work in Theatre Arts, specializing in Oral Traditions and Speech-Interpretation of Literature, with University of Minnesota faculty. She completed a Master of Arts in Education for Gifted, Creative, and Talented Learners with University of St. Thomas faculty and a teaching internship with the International Baccalaureate Program. Her published research, poetry, and drama contribute to the Humanities in Medicine and to the new discipline of Poetry Therapy. Her Chinese calligraphy and brush painting have been exhibited at Trinity Episcopal Cathedral, the Shenzhen Fine Arts Museum in China, and Marylhurst University.

Stephen Rojcewicz, MD, RPT, is a board-certified psychiatrist in private practice in Maryland and a past-president of the National Association for Poetry Therapy. He is fascinated with the integration of mental health, creativity, and the humanities, and has published numerous articles on that theme, as well as papers on suicide and on hallucinations. He is co-author of a textbook on supportive psychotherapy, published by the American Psychiatric Association. He is committed to a greater understanding of other cultures and an ensuing mutual enrichment. Steve also writes poetry and translates poetry from ancient Greek and Latin and several modern languages.

Lily Yueh-Hua Tsang teaches Mandarin Chinese at Journeys of the Heart and the Portland Chinese School. She holds a Master of Arts in Education Curriculum and Instruction from the University of Missouri, Columbia, where she served as assistant principal and teacher for the Columbia Chinese Language School. She holds a Bachelor of Arts in Chinese Literature from Soochow University in Taipei. In addition to teaching and translating, she practices Chinese calligraphy and painting in Hillsboro, Oregon.

Guangying Zhou systematically studied Acupuncture and Chinese Medicine for eleven years at Chengdu University of Traditional Chinese Medicine (TCM), where she earned a doctoral degree in medicine. She has 20 years of clinical experience. Since 1984, she engaged in clinical work, teaching and researching acupuncture and herbal medicine for the Hospital of Chengdu University of TCM, West China University of Medical Sciences, and Sichuan Continuing Educational College of Medical Sciences. She specializes in gynecology and pediatrics. She has successfully treated PMS, various menstrual disorders, menopause syndromes, infertility, acne, digestive disorders, pain syndromes, diabetes, and facial care with acupuncture and herbs. Presently she serves as a visiting professor for the Classical Chinese Medicine Department of the National College of Naturopathic Medicine in Portland, Oregon, where she has taught since 2003. Her scholarly endeavors include directing a series of research projects on menstrual disorders, diabetes, obesity, and anti-senility. She enjoys Chinese calligraphy and Beijing opera.